CONSULTATION-EDUCATION:
DEVELOPMENT AND EVALUATION

Community Mental Health Series

CONSULTATION-EDUCATION
DEVELOPMENT AND EVALUATION

Carole D. Vacher, Ph.D.

Research Psychologist, Division of
Mental Health Services, North Carolina Department of Human Resources

Nicholas E. Stratas, M.D.

Private Practice of Psychiatry; Associate Clinical Professor of Psychiatry,
University of North Carolina; Director
of Physician Education Project

Human Sciences Press
A division of Behavioral Publications
72 Fifth Avenue
New York, New York 10011

Library of Congress Catalog Number 74-19050

ISBN: 0-87705-235-2

Copyright c 1976 by Human Sciences Press,
a division of Behavioral Publications, Inc.,
72 Fifth Avenue, New York, New York 10011

Printed in the United States of America
6789 987654321

TABLE OF CONTENTS

vi

FOREWORD

    The role of the physician in general
practice has long been recognized as a
key position in the total health care
team. The role of continuing education
in enhancing the skills of physicians
and other front line care-giving personnel has more recently gained recognition
as a valuable means of improving the delivery of mental health services.

    As part of the National Institute
of Mental Health's total effort to expand
the mental health resources available
to a community and to improve the quality
of care in mental health services, the
Institute has supported continuing education programs not only for core mental
health disciplines but for all care-giving
personnel in health and related social
welfare programs at State and local levels.

    The Psychiatry-Physician Education
Project directed by Doctor Nicholas E.
Stratas has received continuous NIMH grant

1

support for eight years. It is one of
over 240 continuing education programs
supported since 1966 by the Continuing
Education Branch of NIMH's Division of
Manpower and Training Programs to update
and increase the skills of all those who
serve the mental health needs of their
communities. Of these projects over 100
have been specifically designed to
strengthen the role of the general practice physician in mental health service
delivery.

In this age of rapid social change,
with resultant social-economic-medical
problems, the family physician is often
the first person to whom distraught patients turn even when their problems are
not purely physical. Surveys show that
a large proportion of the patients who
visit general practitioners have an iden-
tifiable mental health problem. The physicians themselves are becoming increas-
ingly aware that they are often the first
to suspect an emotional disorder or illness as they deal with psychological problems related to physical illness.

The family physician, in the best
tradition of medical practice, is concerned not only with the physical health
of his patients, but with their mental
and emotional health as well. Because
of the key position he holds in his community, he is in a unique position not
only to provide mental health services to
his own clientele but to assume a leader-
ship role in helping plan and coordinate
systems of total health care for his community.

Nonpsychiatrist-physicians have often taken the lead in developing mental health services in areas where psychiatry and mental health programs have been nonexistent or have been little understood. Such efforts have proven helpful in preparing a more receptive climate for community mental health planning and the development of mental health service programs.

Two important factors in the rapidly changing mental health picture have given added significance to continuing education in psychiatry for nonpsychiatrist-physicians. First is the advancement of new methods of treatment of mental illness which has resulted in shorter stays for mental patients in mental hospitals and earlier release to home communities for followup treatment and rehabilitation. Second is the rapid expansion of community mental health centers, nursing homes, and other alternatives to hospital care. Both of these factors require the involvement of a wide variety of individuals and groups at the State and local levels, and among the most important are the nonpsychiatrist-physicians who continue their contact with patients through the many components of health care systems.

By expanding the mental health knowledge and skills of physicians and other care-giving individuals who are in the front lines of health care delivery in the community, we can provide better mental health services to all of our people. By disseminating information about training programs, we can stretch the Federal and State dollars to stimulate development of programs in many areas through local and private resources.

Publication of this carefully detailed report on the development and evaluation of this consultation-education project for physicians provides a valuable service to the field. By sharing their experiences, the authors are expanding the impact of this continuing education program. Training program directors can benefit from the process description and evaluation in garnering clues to both positive and negative aspects in developing similar programs. This publication initiated by the project directors helps supplement and expand the project summary published by our Continuing Education Branch in its publication, Continuing Education in Mental Health, and should be of value to all concerned with effective manpower utilization in the field of mental health.

Bertram S. Brown, M.D.
Director
National Institute of Mental Health

ACKNOWLEDGMENTS

We wish to recognize the major contributions of James Cathell, A. R. Mayberry, and Granville Tolley. Doctor James Cathell helped initiate the program and served as co-director and consultant from 1964 until his death in 1969. Doctor A. R. Mayberry joined the program in 1970 and was responsible for expanding the project and building in an evaluation of the entire program. Doctor Granville Tolley provided continuity and direction during the latter part of the project.

We wish to give special acknowledgment to consultants Doctors Charles Vernon, Brooke Johnson, Jesse Cavenar, and the late Bob Martin who permitted us to evaluate their work. We also wish to thank consultants Billy Royal, Roy Clemmons, Harry Johnson, and Jerry Schulte for their contributions during 1971.

Without the support of the North Carolina Department of Mental Health and the encouragement from its members, this

5

project would not have been possible.
The program was funded from January 1964-
June 1966 by the North Carolina Department
of Mental Health. We also wish to extend
our appreciation to the psychiatrists in
the Department who helped verify the questionnaire used in the study.

We are indebted to the National Institute of Mental Health for support from
July 1966-June 1974 through NIMH Grant
MH 10445. During that time Doctor Thomas
Webster and Warren Lamson of the National
Institute of Mental Health were especially
supportive to our program. Doctor Webster
visited the project areas and consulted
with us regarding the development and expansion of the program from 1966-1972.

Many hours were spent consulting with
four professors at North Carolina State
University who served on C. V.'s dissertation committee. We both wish to thank
Doctor Bruce Norton for his counsel regarding the design and conceptual framework parts of the study; Doctor John Wasik
for his assistance with statistical analysis; Doctor Howard Miller who helped us
clarify and elaborate ideas in the method
and results section; and Doctor Paul Marsh
for his understanding and appreciation of
the problems involved in conducting a
program evaluation study.

Before we decided to write the book,
we talked with Doctor Lucy Zabarenko and
Doctor Rex Pittenger of the Staunton Clinic in Pittsburgh. They informed us of
some of the experiences they had while
writing their book on physician education
and encouraged us to share our results
with others.

Invaluable secretarial assistance was provided by Ms. Virginia Woodard who typed several drafts of the manuscript and the final copy of the book. We also thank Ms. Becky Bunn for commenting on some of our earlier drafts. In publishing any material suggestions from editors are very much appreciated. We wish to thank Ms. Norma Fox, Senior Editor of Behavioral Publications, for her useful suggestions during the final stages in the preparation of the book.

INTRODUCTION

The purpose of the book is to share our experiences from 1964-1973 in developing and evaluating a consultation-education program to physicians. The program was first initiated in 1964 in a five county rural area of North Carolina that was noted for its lack of psychiatric resources. In 1967 the program was extended to an urban area of eastern North Carolina and in 1971 to three additional areas of the state. The development of the consultation program and the evaluation of the first phase, 1964-1969, are described in Chapter One.

Additional attention was given to the goals of the program during the second phase, 1970-1973. Assumptions, rationale, theoretical considerations, hypotheses, and evaluation of the second phase of the program are described in Chapter Two. The evaluation that occurred during the second phase sought information about physicians' knowledge, attitudes, and skills. Selection of the sample and

instruments used in collecting data are
presented in Chapter Three. Chapter Four
includes information regarding physician
attitudes toward the mentally ill and
their understanding of etiology, diagnosis, treatment, and referral resources.
This chapter also contains material regarding physicians' hospital referral patterns, drug prescription patterns, attitudes concerning the medical certification process, comfort in working with emotionally disturbed patients, views of
others, discussion of patients' problems
with others, use of community resources,
and time spent with patients.

A summary and conclusions from both
phases of the program are presented in
Chapter Five. The final chapter gives an
account of some of the limitations of the
program and recommendations to other mental health workers who may be interested
in developing or evaluating a consultation
program. We believe that our experiences
can be useful to mental health center
personnel, psychiatrists, social workers,
psychologists, nurses, and other mental
health professionals who may wish to develop a similar program for teachers, ministers, lawyers, police, or other helping
groups. Because consultation was provided
on a one-to-one basis in the individual's
home area, we feel we were successful in
developing a mental health education program that can reach many community groups.

1. FIRST PHASE OF THE CONSULTATION PROGRAM

During the past twenty years, our knowledge of factors contributing to emotional illness and mental health has rapidly increased. We began to focus on methods of preventing mental illness and promoting mental health in addition to the treatment of mental illness. As a result of our increased knowledge about mental health, emphasis on preventive techniques, and awareness of the shortage of mental health personnel to provide treatment services, we examined alternate strategies for meeting the needs of the emotionally disturbed or potentially disturbed individual. Since many individuals turn to physicians, ministers, teachers, or lawyers during periods of stress, we believed that a program designed to teach these community leaders how to identify, recognize, treat, or find an appropriate referral source for the emotionally disturbed would be effective in helping them work with the distressed individual.

Although the program could have been

offered to any of these helping groups,
the focus of the present study was the
family physician. The family physician
is in a strategic position to detect emotional illness even before the individual
himself or his family may be aware of the
problem. He often lives in the community
his entire life and may have known the
individual for several years. In rural
areas the physician may have a close relationship with the individual's family
over two or three generations because of
his presence during births and deaths.
Even the urban physician may have a long-
term understanding of the individual because the physician is the person to whom
many individuals repeatedly turn when they
are in pain. Because the family physician
is in a unique position to detect, prevent,
and treat mental illness, many mental
health education programs have been developed to increase his understanding of psychiatric concepts. Since 1962 the American
Psychiatric Association Committee on Psychiatry and Medical Practice has sponsored
annual colloquiums to further the col-
laboration of psychiatrists and nonpsychiatrist-physicians* in their efforts to prevent mental illness and assist individuals
who have emotional problems. The National
Institute of Mental Health as of 1970,
had spent almost $15,000,000 on psychiatric

---

*The terms nonpsychiatrist-physician, non-
psychiatric-physician, and primary physician have been used to identify practicing
physicians who have not been trained as
psychiatrists. The term nonpsychiatrist-
physician will be used in this book to
identify physicians who participate in
continuing education programs.

education for approximately 11,000 physicians. Two other organizations, the Western Interstate Commission on Higher Education in the western part of the United
States and the Southern Regional Education
Board in the South also have been concerned with developing techniques for making postgraduate psychiatric education
available to physicians since 1960.

The most frequent methods of educating
physicians have been lectures, case discussion methods, small group seminars, and
one- or two-day symposiums. In North
Carolina, seminars and one- or two-day
programs have been conducted by the North
Carolina Department of Mental Health and
the universities in an attempt to educate
the nonpsychiatrist-physician about mental
health. The results of their educative
efforts were no different from other states
who reported that few physicians attended
such programs or that the same group of
physicians were coming year after year.
Green, Hyams, & Haar (1971) estimated that
only ten per cent of all physicians attended such programs. The physician education program that was developed in North
Carolina represented an attempt to educate
an even greater percentage of physicians
about mental health concepts. The program
was not developed with the intent of replacing lectures, case discussion methods,
seminars, or symposiums, but represented
another educational approach for teaching
physicians about mental health concepts.

DEVELOPMENT OF A MENTAL HEALTH PROGRAM
FOR FAMILY PHYSICIANS IN NORTH CAROLINA

Before 1963 mental health services
in North Carolina were organized through
a governor-appointed Hospitals Board of
Control that was primarily concerned with
the treatment of emotionally disturbed
individuals in four mental hospitals in
the state. A small community mental
health program was administered by the
Board of Health. In 1963 legislation was
passed to create the North Carolina Department of Mental Health which was given
the authority to develop a wide range program for the prevention and treatment of
mental illness. Special attention was
given to providing care for the emotionally disturbed individual in his home community. Part of the appropriation from
the legislature included funds for the
positions of a state-wide Director of
Professional Education and Training and
a Director of Community Services. The
position of Director of Professional Education and Training was filled by one of
the authors of the book. A psychiatrist
who was appointed Director of Community
Services had formerly been responsible
for developing continuing education programs for physicians throughout the state.
These two individuals and the Commissioner
of Mental Health, a strong advocate of
educational programs, began discussing
possible types of mental health education
programs that would meet the needs of the
emotionally disturbed in the state.

During this same period the Director
of Professional Education and Training had

been working with a psychiatrist who was
serving as director of the aftercare clinic in one of the state mental hospitals.
They discussed the possibility of developing a mental health education program
for physicians in the western part of
the state where few or no psychiatric resources existed. Discussions among this
psychiatrist, the Commissioner, the Director of Community Services, and the Director of Education and Training provided
the basis for the idea of educating one
family physician in each western county
to become a mental health resource person
for other physicians residing in the county. Since past experiences in providing
seminars for physicians at the university
had not been too successful, these individuals believed that a program in which
a psychiatrist would travel to visit the
physician in his home community might be
better received. The psychiatrist who
lived in the western part of the state
was employed to visit with physicians and
help develop a mental health education
program for them. Funds for this psychiatrist's position were obtained initially
from an unfilled physician position at
the state mental hospital in the western
part of the state. In 1966 the program
was funded by the National Institute of
Mental Health.

     Members of the State Medical Society
had been instrumental in passing legislation that created the State Department of
Mental Health because they believed the
Department could help provide additional
mental health resources to counties
throughout the state. North Carolina
Department of Mental Health personnel felt

it was necessary to obtain sanction from
the State Medical Society before initiating the mental health education program to
physicians residing in the western counties. They were able to obtain that support through the influence of local medical societies in the western part of the
state.

A decision was made to begin the
program in several rural counties in the
western part of the state after the two
project co-directors were named. One co-
director was responsible for the organi-
zation and development of the program and
the second for consultation to physicians
in the western part of the state.

The first step in initiating the
program was to identify the counties to
be served by the program. After the co-
directors examined the 31-county area con-
taining a population of over 500,000 people, they realized that they could not
offer the program to all of them at first.
The co-directors decided to extend the
program to only 16 counties in the north-
western part of the state that had few,
if any, psychiatric resources.

The scope of the program was nar-
rowed, but the goals of identifying one
physician who could be trained as a mental
health resource person and in turn teach
other physicians about mental health concepts remained the same. The next step
was to contact physicians in these 16
western counties. A letter was sent to
the president and the chairman of the mental health committee of each medical society, inviting them to a meeting at the

state hospital in the western part of the
state to discuss mental health resources
in their counties. The letters were followed by telephone calls to the presi-
dents and chairmen of the mental health
committee of each medical society.

Sixty physicians instead of the six-
teen expected to attend came to the meeting. The group was informed that a psychiatrist was available to serve as a
psychiatric consultant to the 16 counties
if there was a physician in each county
who wished to participate. The Super-
intendent of the State Mental Hospital
in the western area was also present at
the meeting and opened the discussion by
stating that physicians were needed to
help with patients returning to their
home communities. Several of the 60 physicians who attended the meeting stated
that they were currently seeing many patients who had been released from the
hospital and were keeping many patients
out of the hospital. They expressed an
interest in receiving mental health information from the consultant in addition
to information on dealing with the aftercare patient. They wanted to know how
to successfully treat emotional problems
of patients who may not need the services
of a mental hospital. All of the sixty
physicians who attended the meeting expressed a wish to be involved in the psychiatric consultation program rather than
selecting only one physician from each
of their counties to receive the services
of the psychiatric consultant. In fact,
the physicians suggested that the psychiatric consultant visit all of the 16
counties and meet with them either in

groups or individually. As a result of
the interest and suggestions made by the
60 physicians who attended the meetings,
the co-directors decided to visit each of
the county medical societies before making
any additional plans.

After meetings were held with the
medical societies in each of the local
counties, a pilot project was begun in
only four of the counties* instead of the
16, since there was no way of estimating
the amount of time the consultant would
need to spend with each physician.

The four counties initially selected
for the pilot project contained a very
disperse rural population of 130,000 individuals. Alleghany County (population
8,000) had six physicians and a 50-bed
general hospital. Ashe County (population
20,000) also had a 50-bed hospital and six
physicians. Two hospitals (100 beds and
32 beds) and 12 physicians were located in
Avery County (population 12,000). Watauga
County (population 20,000) had nine physicians and two hospitals (91 beds and 32
beds, later enlarged to 103 beds). The
next year, a fifth county was added. Cald-
well (population 50,000) had 33 physicians
and three hospitals (32 beds, 140 beds,
and 50 beds). None of the counties had
either a psychiatrist, a mental health
clinic, or provision for local psychiatric
hospitalization. Psychiatric consultation
was provided to 65 of the 68 physicians
in these five counties from 1964 through
1967.

---

*A fifth county was added in 1965.

STAGES IN THE CONSULTATION PROCESS

The co-director was not aware of definite stages in the consultation program at the time it was developing, but he identified five stages in the consultation process after working with physicians for one, two, or three years. The stages were: entry, testing and orientation, dependence, premature independence, and interdependence. Each stage will be identified as the program is discussed.

The actual implementation of the program in the four pilot counties began at the time the co-directors obtained information about the community and its power structure. The co-directors visited with representatives of the school system and welfare and health departments. They also talked with service station attendants, funeral directors, pharmacists, and other residents of the counties in order to learn about community resources and identify key decision-makers in the communities and among the physicians themselves. The co-director who was providing the consultation was familiar to the people residing in the western counties because he had lived there for several years. Physicians believed he understood their problems since he had previously worked as a general practitioner for 11 years.

I. Entry

The purpose of the initial visit to each physician was to establish a working relationship and arrange a scheduled time to meet. Some physicians expressed a desire to meet during regular office hours, others asked for meetings at the local hospital during morning or evening rounds, and a few preferred to meet during mealtimes or around some recreational activity. The consultant told physicians that his role was not to provide direct treatment services to patients but to discuss ways of helping them deal with emotionally disturbed patients. He also informed them that there was no fee for his services. The psychiatrist felt it necessary to clarify his role with them at first in order to reduce any fears the physicians may have had regarding a financial obligation to him, or feelings that he was attempting to change their style of practice.

Most of the physicians he contacted initially scheduled regular times for him to visit. Other physicians were not interested in seeing the consultant at a regular time, and in these instances, the consultant visited the physician again during his regular practice hours. Because of the varied schedules of the physician, the consultant discovered that he needed to maintain a very flexible schedule. It took approximately eight months to work out a regular schedule of visits to each physician. The consultant gave all the physicians his weekly schedule and told them he was available by phone

if they needed to contact him during a
nonscheduled visit. Other physicians did
not participate in the program at first
and waited until they were faced with a
crisis before seeking the consultant's
assistance. Traditionally physicians have
referred a patient to another physician
for a consultation regarding diagnosis or
recommendations for treatment. Oftentimes
it was necessary to inform the physicians
that the consultation provided in this
program differed from consultation employed by specialists in a hospital set-
ting because the psychiatric consultant
preferred to discuss the patient's problem
with the physician rather than diagnosing
or treating the patient himself. The consultation employed in this program also
differed from that described by Caplan
(1970). Caplan sees the consultee as in-
voking the consultant's help in regard to
a problem with which he is having difficulty. In this program the consultant
was presented to the physician as a mental health resource person representing
the Department of Mental Health and having
obtained the support of the local medical
societies for the service he was providing
to the physicians. The sanction of the
two groups helped establish his credibility and facilitate his efforts in estab-
lishing his role with the physicians.

II. *Testing and Orientation*

The next stage in the consultation
process usually occurred after the consultant's second, third, or fourth visit.
This was a testing and orientation phase

because physicians had arranged for the
consultant to see several of their most
difficult patients. These were often the
physician's most chronically complaining
patients. Some of the physicians expected
the consultant to see the patient and
make recommendations, and others expected
the consultant to treat the patient himself. Although the consultant's original
purpose was to discuss the patient and
make recommendations to the physician,
in some cases he believed it would help
establish the confidence of the physician
if he saw the patient. He saw some of the
patients with the physician in his office
and again told him his chief purpose was
to make recommendations instead of treating a patient. Although these were the
physicians' worst patients, we believed
this was a testing of the consultant. The
situation also provided the consultant
with an opportunity to demonstrate his
competence in interviewing, diagnosing,
and treating the mentally disturbed person.

During this same phase, opportunities
arose for the consultant to be supportive
to the physician in the work he had begun
with these difficult patients. He was
able to help the physician generalize his
learnings to other patients who had similar problems. As the physician talked
about particularly difficult patients the
consultant was often able to help him
recognize and accept angry and guilty
feelings that may have prevented him from
being effective with the patient. Through
the support and confidence of the consultant, the physician was able to find alternate ways of working with the patient.

Patient goals were frequently reviewed
with the physicians, and idealistic or
theoretical goals were converted to more
realistic expectations. This was particularly the case with alcoholic or drug
patients. For instance, instead of curing
the alcoholic, a more appropriate goal
might be to detoxify the acute alcoholic
and arrange for family or other agency
support. Throughout this stage the consultant was willing to see patients with
the physicians if he perceived that continuation of the relationship was dependent upon it.

III. Dependence

At this stage the physicians had become very confident of the consultant's
ability to work with disturbed patients
and waited for his opinion before making
independent judgements regarding a patient. During this stage the consultant
began decreasing his involvement with
clients and began helping consultees real-
ize they were responsible for patient
improvement. At first he asked the consultee to observe while he interviewed
the patient, later he observed while the
physician interviewed the patient, and
finally he moved to a discussion of the
case with the consultee. In this stage
the consultee began to ask questions concerning history and diagnosis and presented cases other than their so-called
"crocks" to the consultant. This was the
busiest phase for the consultant. It was
at this stage that the consultee first
initiated telephone contact with the

consultant. This "dependent" stage ended
as the consultee saw that he was not only
responsible for patient improvement, but
also had acquired significant new information.

IV. Premature Independence

During stage IV, the physicians became somewhat prematurely independent.
The consultee felt so successful that he
sometimes had greater expectations of himself than he could fulfill. Physicians
began discussing fewer patients with the
consultant, making fewer telephone contacts, and distancing themselves somewhat
from the consultant. They shifted from
stating "what shall I do" to "this is what
I have done." The physician often took
on cases which he was not prepared to handle, and the consultant was forced to wait
until the consultee requested his assistance after a failure. The physician
once again became temporarily dependent
on the consultant for the cases he had
mismanaged. Those who had difficulty during this stage reached the final stage
more quickly than the others.

V. Interdependence

In the last stage the consultant and
the physician were more interdependent
because they exchanged ideas on the appropriate handling of the case. The consultee had confidence in his ability to
work effectively with the patient, while

the consultant supported the consultee in
his ability to function independently.
Consultees and consultants used their time
most efficiently in this stage because
they were able to discuss more patients in
a short period of time. Consultees began
to seek the consultant's advice more often
by telephone. The focus of the consultation shifted from requests for assistance
with diagnosis to emphasis on treatment.

EVALUATION OF FIRST PHASE
OF CONSULTATION PROGRAM

The co-directors believed the consultation program had been effective in
teaching physicians about mental health
concepts, but they needed some objective
measurement of this effectiveness. In
1968 they contacted the Director of the
Social Science Research Institute of North
Carolina who informed them it was too late
to conduct a thorough evaluation, but a
postevaluation might provide some mean-
ingful information. Hallman and Havey
(1969), two researchers at the Institute,
interviewed some of the physicians who
had participated in the project from 1964-
1967 and obtained information about the
program and the consultant.

The consultees reported that the
consultant had been most helpful in the
areas of interviews, diagnosis, treatment, and prescription of appropriate
drugs for the disturbed patient. He was
also seen as a very valuable resource
during the times physicians found it necessary to commit a patient to the state

hospital or wanted a feedback regarding a patient they had referred to the mental hospital. The consultant helped physicians decide if they could maintain patients in their home communities with supportive therapy or drug treatment or whether commitment to the hospital was necessary. Since the consultant initially served as Director of the state hospital's outpatient clinic, he was able to report on the progress of the patients the physicians had referred to the mental hospital.

Physicians also found the consultant helpful because of the emotional support he gave them in working with difficult patients. They reported that he was particularly supportive to the physician in dealling with legal or ethical issues and discussing commitment procedures with the patients' families.

Several of the consultees reported that they believed the personality of the consultant was an important factor contributing to the success of the program. He was described as "a special type of person," "a rustic person," "not in an ivory tower," and "easy to talk to." Some consultees thought that the program was successful because of the consultant's knowledge of psychiatric concepts. Others thought he was able to understand their particular problems because of his previous experience as a general practitioner. Another factor that physicians identified as important to the success of the program was the consultant's commitment to his task. Physicians perceived him as "wanting to help us," "desiring to help the patient

first," and "liking the work and wanting
to do it."

The interviewers concluded that the
factors responsible for the physicians'
acceptance of the consultation program were
the consultant's (1) patience and skill in
allowing the consultee to progress through
five stages of development, and (2) the
ability of the consultant to support the
consultee while trying new skills.   Although a large part of the consultant's
role was educative, most of his time and
energy was devoted to developing and maintaining relationships with the consultee
that would permit him to learn about mental
health concepts.

The interviewers also asked the physicians about the type of drugs they used
with the emotionally disturbed patient.
They were interested in knowing what drugs,
dose range, and combination of drugs physicians used for specific emotional disorders, and in what instances these drugs
were prescribed.   The interviewers desired
this type of information because the consultant had noted that physicians often
(1) would not give a drug sufficient time
to take effect before prescribing another
drug, (2) would change the prescription
the state hospital aftercare clinic had
prescribed for a patient, (3) would give
inadequate dosages of phenothiazines, and
(4) would give patients the manufacturer's
latest drug samples although they were
unfamiliar with them.   Physicians reported
that they found the drug information delivered by the consultant helpful.   The
interviewers concluded that following consultation the physicians (1) did not switch

drugs that were originally prescribed by
state hospital physicians for aftercare
patients, (2) used few psychoactive drug
combinations, (3) used high dosages of the
phenothiazines rather than a high dosage
of a minor tranquilizer to treat the severely disturbed individual, and (4) allowed a period of one to two weeks for the
antidepressant medication to take effect.

Since evaluation of the program was
conducted after the program terminated in
the five western counties, it did not provide much information on the program's
effectiveness in improving the physicians'
knowledge of mental health and changing
their attitudes and skills toward the
mentally ill. One measure of effectiveness
was obtained by examining the number of
psychiatric admissions to the state mental
hospital and local general hospitals in
the area. It was expected that the number
of psychiatric admissions to the general
hospitals would increase and admissions to
the state hospital would decrease as physicians became aware of the importance of
keeping the emotionally disturbed patient
close to his home community where he could
obtain support from family and friends.
The psychiatric consultant (co-director)
asked local hospital administrators to
examine the types of admissions to their
hospitals during the fiscal year 1962-
1963--the year before the project began--
and during the years 1964-1966 while the
consultation program was in effect in the
western part of the state. Although re-
porting was done verbally, hospital administrators in the original four-county area
stated that the number of psychiatric
admissions increased from 10 per cent in

1962-1963 to 30 per cent in 1965-1966.
Psychiatric admissions to the state mental
hospital in the original four counties
served by the consultation program were
compared with two areas that did not receive consultation. One area contained
two counties that had mental health clinics in operation during the period consultation was employed and another area consisted of four counties that had no psychiatric resources. Data obtained during
the first two years of the program showed
that admissions decreased by 30 per cent
in the four-county area receiving consultation while they increased in the two
areas that did not have access to the consultation program. Admissions increased
by 15 per cent in the adjacent four-county
area that had no mental health resources
and by 42 per cent in the area that had
two mental health clinics. The decrease
in the number of psychiatric admissions to
the state mental hospitals and increase in
psychiatric admissions to local general
hospitals indicated the program was successful in teaching physicians to use local
community resources for the treatment of
the emotionally disturbed patient.

Another indication of program effectiveness was obtained by examining readmissions to the state mental hospital in
the areas served by the project and in the
areas that did not receive consultation.
The greatest number occurred in the area
that did not have access to consultation.
In the area that did not receive consultation and did not have any mental health
resources, readmissions increased by 50
per cent. An increase of 22 per cent was
noted in the two-county area that did not

have access to consultation but had two
mental health clinics. Readmissions increased by only 13 per cent in the counties receiving consultation. These percentages indicate that the consultation
program was successful in the area receiving consultation because physicians
who had received consultation were able
to either treat the discharged mental patient in their offices or find another
local community resource for him instead
of readmitting him to the state hospital.

CONSULTATION TO PHYSICIANS IN
THE EASTERN PART OF THE STATE

As a result of the success of the
consultation program in a rural area,
members of the North Carolina Department
of Mental Health were interested in determining if the same type of program could
be applied in an urban area of the state.
The original goal of the North Carolina
Department of Mental Health was to extend
the program to all four regions of the
state, North Carolina is divided into
four geographic regions for mental health
services. A state mental hospital located
in each of these regions serves the population of the region (see map, Appendix
A).

In mid-1967 the consultation program
was begun in New Hanover County in which
Wilmington, a city of 50,000, is located,
In New Hanover County there were three
hospitals comprising a total bed capacity
of 479. One was a general hospital con-
taining a 12-bed psychiatric unit, another

the state's only pediatric hospital, and
the third, a general hospital. In addition to the hospital resources there
were three psychiatrists in private practice plus 85 physicians in the area. The
rural counties of Pender (population
28,000) and Brunswick (population 22,000)
were served by the mental health clinic
in that area and were also selected to
receive consultation from the psychiatric
consultant. Pender County had a 47-bed
general hospital and Brunswick County a
50-bed general hospital. Each county had
four physicians.

Psychiatric consultation in the two
eastern rural counties was similar to that
conducted in the western rural counties
although more psychiatric facilities were
available to the physicians in the eastern
counties. All eight of the practicing
physicians in the two rural counties participated in the consultation program.
Although no interviews were conducted with
the physicians who participated in the
program in the east, the psychiatric consultant (co-director) reported that the
physicians in the east went through the
same succession of stages as the physicians in the western part of the state,
and 14 of the 39 with whom he worked
reached the stage of interdependence after
a year. The psychiatric consultant (co-
director) believed he was most helpful
to physicians in the eastern part of the
state because he was available to fill in
some of the nonexisting psychiatric resources. Since there was no child psychiatrist in the area, he fulfilled this
need by consulting with pediatricians and
moving his office from the mental health

clinic to Babies' Hospital (a children's hospital). Physicians found his services useful in helping them decide which patients needed or would most likely benefit from a psychiatric referral. He believed he was helpful because he was almost always immediately available to physicians when they needed him.

The consultant found it necessary to change his consultation style to physicians in the urban area of Wilmington because there was a greater ratio of physicians to the population, fewer primary care physicians than specialists, and the total number of physicians was greater than the number with which he had previously worked in the western counties. Instead of scheduling regular meetings with physicians once or twice a month, he attended hospital staff meetings and specialty conferences held once or twice monthly. He believed that attendance at these meetings would alert physicians to his availability and the resources he could provide them. He avoided regularly scheduled meetings with urban physicians because there were too many of them to visit individually, and specialist physicians did not want to spend time in individual consultation. Specialist physicians were interested in a brief consultation around a specific area rather than general knowledge about mental health, and some physicians were not motivated to help some patients who had mental health problems because of the availability of psychiatric resources. The consultant observed that physicians who were specialists, usually located in an urban area, expected a more traditional type of

consultation because their problems were
more crisis oriented, fewer patients were
discussed, and the relationship with them
was less intense. In contrast, primary
care physicians, especially the physician
located in a rural area, seemed to accept
responsibility for patients with many
types of problems because there were limited resources for referral. The consultant believed that practicing physicians
in a rural area needed consultation in
more general areas and may require a more
involved and longer term relationship
with the consultant.

At this point the total project was
re-examined. It was recognized that specific goals must be identified, steps
toward achieving these goals initiated,
and that the project be expanded to more
than two areas. The next chapter de-
scribes the changes that occurred as a
clearer design and evaluation were imple-
mented.

REFERENCES

Caplan, G. *The theory and practice of mental
      health consultation.* New York: Basic
      Books, 1970.
Green, M. R., Hyams, L. & Harr, E.   Inter-
      actional problems between mental
      health professionals, and non-psy-
      chiatric physicians. *Mental Hygiene,*
      1971, *55*   (2),206-213.
Hallman, S. P. & Havey, T. G.   *Psychiatric
      education of general practitioners through
      consultation: an exploratory study.*   Chap-
      el Hill, North Carolina: Social

Research Section of the Division of
Health Affairs, 1969.

2. SECOND PHASE OF THE CONSULTATION PROGRAM

During 1964-1969, physicians who participated in the consultation program and community leaders residing in counties where the program was employed told North Carolina Department of Mental Health personnel that they thought the program was successful and hoped that it could continue. Some physicians who participated in the consultation program believed it was successful because of the particular characteristics and style of the consultant. Members of the North Carolina Department of Mental Health and the co-director of the project recognized the contributions of the original psychiatric consultant but contended that other individuals could also be successful consultants. Because of these beliefs a decision was made to expand the program to additional areas of the state after the original psychiatric consultant's death in 1969. Goals and scope of the program were modified after a new psychiatric consultant (co-director) was employed in 1970. The new psychiatric consultant (co-director)

35

had formerly served as Clinical Director
of a mental health center for several
years, where he had consulted with physicians and taught them to use community resources. He was interested in re-examining
the goals of the program, extending the
program to several areas of the state, and
evaluating the effectiveness of the program. During the early months of 1971,
the new psychiatric co-director employed
six psychiatrists and one psychologist to
conduct consultation in five areas of the
state (see map, Appendix A). Since evaluation of the 1964-1967 phase of the program was conducted after the program was
in operation and did not provide the consultant with information regarding effectiveness of the consultation, he wanted
to build in an evaluation of the second
phase of the program from the beginning.
A research psychologist was employed to
design an evaluation of the program.

In an attempt to find a design and
instruments that would best measure the
effectiveness of the consultation program,
the literature on consultation and training programs to nonpsychiatrist-physicians
was reviewed. A very complete review of
the literature on training programs to
general practitioners was reported by
Zabarenko et al (1968) and a review of the
consultation literature by Bindman (1966),
and Mannino and Shore (1971). A review
of only the evaluative studies on consultation and mental health training programs
to physicians was reported by Vacher
(1973). These studies are summarized
below.

Most of the studies related to training of general practitioners have been descriptive. Small group seminars, case conferences, lectures, long-term courses, and supervised clinical experiences have been used to educate the nonpsychiatrist-physician. The goals of most of these programs have been to increase the doctor's understanding of the emotional needs of his patients and to improve the doctor-patient relationship. The content of the courses has focused on teaching principles of conducting an interview, and methods of diagnosis, treatment, and rehabilitation. Evaluation of these courses has often been subjective consisting only of verbal reports by instructors of what they think participants have learned. Others have used interviews, intensive observations over long periods of time, case studies, pre-existing questionnaires, reactions to filmed and recorded interviews, and objectively scored tests. Some researchers have devised their own instruments to measure effectiveness of the courses. Most have attempted to assess changes in psychiatric concepts and attitudes after the course, or measure changes in attitudes in working with patients.

These studies have identified characteristics of those physicians who do well in seminar type instruction and characteristics of physicians who change their attitudes. Unfortunately, incomplete description of the instruments used to obtain the data, and poorly defined criteria for judging the effectiveness of the program presented problems in generalizing information to another population. Moreover, results of the evaluation of these

brief courses suggested little real effect
occurred in changing knowledge or improving attitudes of participants. Two of the
studies reported that physicians who participated in the courses for additional
periods of time improved the most.

Bindman (1966) and Mannino & Shore
(1971) found many studies describing consultation activities in several fields,
but very few were empirical. Mannino &
Shore (1971) state that research in consultation is plagued with many of the same
problems as psychotherapy, but is even
more difficult because the definition of
consultation and its goals are less well
defined and target groups reside in many
settings. Most studies have not concep-
tualized the variables studied, have not
had hypotheses to test, have lacked control groups, have not referred to previous
studies on consultation, and have not been
replicated.

Evaluative studies on consultation to
schools, public health departments, police
departments, neighborhood service centers,
and community agencies were reviewed. Instruments for assessing change have ranged
from a simple subjective evaluation to
observation by teachers, intensive before-
and-after interviews by the physician participants, and objective scales and tests.
Length of time and quality of the relationship between the consultant and the
consultee appeared to be important factors
in producing change in the consultee. Although strict designs for these studies
have not been impressive, results of these
evaluative studies have indicated that

consultees found their consultation experiences favorable.

Few evaluative studies were found
in the area of consultation and even fewer
in the area of mental health training programs to physicians. We did not find any
evaluative studies on psychiatric consultation programs to physicians. More evaluative studies are needed in order to develop a theory of consultation. Mannino
& Shore (1971) state that crisis theory,
ecologic theory, and systems theory could
supply a useful orientation to consultation, but currently none of these has
gained acceptance.

After reviewing the literature and
reflecting upon some of the errors of
omission that occurred during the planning
and evaluation of the first phase of the
project, more attention was given to the
rationale and assumptions of the program
during the second phase. First, formal
hypotheses were stated and second, instruments were designed or obtained to measure
knowledge, attitudes, and skills acquired
by physicians participating in the program. Since no one theory of consultation
had gained wide acceptance, it was believed that a theory that might offer some
explanation of how the consultation process operated would be useful to those
interested in consultation. The rationale, assumptions, hypotheses, theoretical
considerations, and a chronological description of events that occurred during
the second phase are presented in this
chapter.

RATIONALE

A major reason for evaluation of the consultation program was to determine its effectiveness in educating physicians about mental health concepts. Van Matre (1964) reviewed the federal funding of postgraduate education in psychiatry and noted that in 1958 the Senate Appropriations Committee made a special allocation of $1,300,000 for the basic psychiatric instruction of physicians. From fiscal year 1959 through 1963, 239 grants totaling $3,446,419 were made to 70 institutions for psychiatric education to practicing physicians. Lamson (1974) of the National Institute of Mental Health reported that grants totaled as much as $1,114,832 in fiscal year 1963. Several programs have evaluated the effectiveness of their efforts, but very few have conducted comprehensive and in depth evaluations of the overall program.

Another reason for the study, although not the original purpose, was to examine some theoretical concepts that might help explain the consultation process. In May 1971, after the second phase of the program had begun and the research design developed, we became aware of our failure to plan our design upon any theoretical base. Since no one theory of consultation had gained acceptance, it was decided to examine some of the concepts of learning theory in order to determine if this theory might provide some framework from which to base our assumptions and hypotheses. Theories of reinforcement have been successfully applied to explain numerous events in the laboratory but have not satisfactorily explained events that occur in the community. The present study was concerned with determining if a laboratory theory could partially explain some of the events that occurred during the consultation process.

ASSUMPTIONS

The first phase of the consultation program operated on the assumption that consultation as a technique for educating physicians about mental health was superior to the lecture or case seminar method. Consultation in which the consultant visited with the consultee individually in his office or work area was seen as a vehicle for reaching some of the often quoted 90 per cent of nonpsychiatrist-physicians who did not participate in continuing education programs.

During the second phase of the project, additional thought was given to providing a theoretical framework for some of these assumptions. We believed that learning of mental health concepts could occur best in a one-to-one relationship in which the consultant could provide verbal reinforcement to the physician for new or currently existing behaviors. Although the present study was not designed to test this assumption, it was believed that behavior change could occur in physicians by verbal reinforcement from the consultant. Greenspoon (1955) demonstrated that subjects increased in the frequency of plural responses when the experimenter said "mmm-hmm" and decreased in plural responses when "uh-huh" was said. Several studies have shown that behaviors can be modified in this way. Hildum & Brown (1956) found that saying "good" was a sufficient reinforcer to modify attitudes on an issue although "mm-hmm" was not. Ekman (1958) found that saying "good" and the nonverbal nod and smile were equally effective. Singer (1961) found that saying "good" or "right" by the examiner each time subjects agreed with pro-democratic statements produced a change in attitudes toward a more "democratic" position.

A verbal reinforcer can be expected to be more effective when delivered by a person whom the subject views as an expert or with whom he wishes to identify. Krasner et al (1965) found that verbal reinforcement ("good" and "hmm-mm") delivered by an "expert" could shift attitudes toward medical science in a favorable, but not unfavorable direction.

These studies and many others uncited have shown that attitude statements can be increased or modified by verbal reinforcement. It is believed that future researchers might find this theory particularly useful in studying the consultation process.

THEORETICAL CONSIDERATIONS

Learning theory approaches have been applied to the social situations of language acquisition, imitative behavior,

attitude formation and change, behavior
change in psychotherapy, the socialization
process, judgment of self and others, and
group interaction. The reinforcement theory of attitude change is used in the present study as a means of understanding some
of the forces operating to bring about
change in physicians as a result of consultation. Instrumental learning or reinforcement theory approaches to attitude
acquisition are based on the notion that
attitudes consist of overt verbal behavior.
Attitudes can be taught by varying reinforcement contingencies so as to shape the
desired behavior. Cohen (1964) reports
that who says something is as important
as what is said in producing attitude
change. He asserts that the vividness of
the communicator's person, his status, and
the expertise attributed to him can affect
the way the listener perceives the communicator. Studies varying the occupation
or role of the communicator with his degree of expertness have been conducted by
Hovland & Weiss (1951), Kelman & Hovland
(1953), Bergin (1962), Aronson et al
(1963), and Choo (1964). They reported
that attitude change was greatest in subjects who received communications from a
highly credible communicator. Aronson
et al (1963) and Choo (1964) found that
the high credibility source produced more
attitude change than the low credibility
source even among subjects who viewed the
communication as discrepant from their own
position.

On the basis of these studies this
study assumes that physician perception
of the consultant as an expert or prestigious person will be responsible for

producing change in physician knowledge, attitudes, and performance skills.

ASSUMPTIONS ABOUT CURRENT BEHAVIORS OF PHYSICIANS

Caplan (1970, p. 127) states that consultee-centered consultation is employed when there is (1) lack of knowledge, (2) lack of skill, (3) lack of self confidence, and (4) lack of professional objectivity. He states that the nonpsychiatrist-physician's inability to handle patients with emotional problems may be due to his lack of knowledge about psychosocial factors. Caplan maintains that courses in psychology, psychopathology, community mental health, and the areas of alcoholism, drug addiction, suicide, mental retardation, and crisis theory have been neglected in medical school training. This is especially true of the older practitioner.

According to instrumental learning theory, subjects' responses are instrumental in securing the reinforcer which in turn increases the frequency of the response; therefore, any change in physician behavior must be due to reinforcement of that behavior. In order to determine which rewards or incentives will operate to change physician behavior, one must first identify the current behaviors of the physicians.

In this project our assumptions about physician behavior were that physicians were uncomfortable in working with the

emotionally disturbed patient because of
their lack of knowledge about mental health
and mental illness, unfavorable attitudes
toward the mentally ill person, and poor
skills in dealing with the emotionally
disturbed patient.

HYPOTHESES

The assumptions we made in the last
section led to the following hypotheses.

Hypothesis I: Physician Knowledge Would
                   Change

                   Ia: Experimental physicians'
                   scores on the case studies would
                   be significantly higher than
                   control physicians' scores.

In order to determine if physician
knowledge had increased, physicians were
presented with five case studies (see
Appendix C) and asked to respond to questions regarding (a) etiology, (b) clinical
impression, (c) diagnostic approach,
(d) treatment, and (e) referral source
for the emotionally disturbed patient. We
believed that physicians could be taught
to recognize mental illness which might
first appear disguised as physical illness.
Physician achievement was determined by
comparing pre- and post-scores in these
five areas. It was expected that physicians receiving consultation would score
significantly higher on the post-questionnaire because they would have acquired new
information regarding etiology, clinical

impression, diagnostic approach, treatment approach, and referral resources for the emotionally disturbed individual from the information delivered by the consultant.

Hypothesis II: Physicians' Attitudes
Would Change

One measure of physician attitudes was obtained from scores on the social distance and social responsibility attitude scale (see Appendix C). Additional attitudinal measures were obtained from responses to items on the interview schedule (see Appendix D).

> IIa: Experimental physicians
> would obtain significantly
> lower scores than controls on
> social distance and higher
> scores on social responsibility.

We expected that experimental physicians would increase in attitudes of social responsibility and decrease in attitudes of social distance toward the mentally ill as they gained an understanding from the consultant of some of the factors responsible for mental illness and acquired new skills in working with these individuals. The assumption underlying this hypothesis was that physicians might wish to identify with the consultant and adopt his values of acceptance and tolerance toward the mentally ill.

> IIb: Experimental physicians
> would report significantly more
> times than control physicians
> that they felt more comfortable

in working with the psychiatric
patient after consultation.

Physicians generally feel comfortable
in working with patients in areas in which
they have had specific training. Since
two of the goals of the consultation program were to provide new understanding
about mental health and mental illness and
support to the physician in working with
the emotionally disturbed, it was expected
they would report feeling more comfortable
in working with the emotionally disturbed
patient after consultation.

IIc: Experimental physicians
would report significantly more
times than controls that they
viewed nurses, office workers,
and medical colleagues differently after consultation.

As physicians acquired greater understanding of mental health concepts, we
believed they might begin to apply these
learnings to individuals with whom they
worked.

IId: Experimental physicians
would report significantly more
times than control physicians
that they perceived the medical
certification process for admitting patients to mental hospitals as less cumbersome after
participating in the program.

We contended that it was possible
physicians viewed commitment procedures
to the mental hospital as difficult because they did not know personnel at the

hospital or procedures that would make commitment easier when it was necessary. Consultants might relieve the physician of the assumption that hospitalization was the only alternative available to the mentally ill person, or physicians might learn about other community resources that could be of service to the emotionally disturbed person.

Hypothesis III: Physician Skills
                    Would Change

Information regarding current skills of the physician was obtained by examining experimental and control group interview responses (see Appendix D) concerning drug prescription patterns, referrals to community resources, and discussion of patients who had emotional problems. The number and types of referrals to the mental hospitals and mental health centers were obtained by examining physician referral patterns to these resources the year before consultation began and the year consultation was in effect.

> IIIa: Experimental physicians would decrease significantly from 1971 to 1972 in the total number of psychiatric referrals and in the total number of alcoholic and geriatric referrals to mental hospitals. Experimental physicians would increase significantly from 1971 to 1972 in the total number of psychiatric referrals and total number of alcoholic and geriatric referrals to the

mental health centers. No significant differences were expected among the control group
from 1971 to 1972 in the total
number of referrals to mental
hospitals or mental health centers.

One of the goals of the consultation
program was to inform physicians about the
importance of utilizing community resources
and personnel in providing total care for
the emotionally disturbed patient. As experimental physicians became aware of the
importance of maintaining the individual
in his home community where he could obtain
support from family and friends, we believed that they would decrease in their
total number of referrals to mental hospitals. Consultants had identified alcoholic
and geriatric patients as two groups on
which they would focus their consultative
efforts. We expected that experimental
physicians would learn about community resources or acquire methods of dealing with
these patients in their offices rather than
referring them to the mental hospital.

IIIb: Experimental physicians
would report that they prescribed
significantly more times than
controls (1) major tranquilizers,
antidepressants, and fewer barbiturates for the severely disturbed patient, and (2) more
minor tranquilizers and fewer
barbiturates for the mildly disturbed patient or individual in
a crisis situation.

The consultants' previous experiences in working with community physicians led them to believe that many nonpsychiatrist-physicians tended to prescribe too few major tranquilizers and too many barbiturates for the emotionally disturbed individual. They thought that the nonpsychiatrist-physician needed to learn to differentiate between antipsychotic, antianxiety, and antidepressant drugs and how to prescribe appropriate dosages for the type of disorder the individual presented.

> IIIc: Experimental physicians would report that they referred significantly more patients to public health departments, private psychiatrists, mental health centers, family service agencies, child guidance or developmental evaluation clinics, alcoholics anonymous, and welfare departments during 1972 than did control physicians.

One of the goals of the program was to inform physicians about existing community resources and the advantages of local treatment for the patient when possible. Consultants reported that many of the physicians in their communities were not using local resources available to them.

> IIId: Experimental physicians would report a significantly greater frequency of instances than controls, that they discussed patients who had emotional problems with medical colleagues, local ministers,

members of the patient's family,
school personnel, and hospital
personnel.

After physicians learned about the
importance of involving others in planning total patient care, it was expected
they would discuss with family, medical
colleagues, hospital personnel, ministers,
and school personnel how they could be of
support to the patient during and following his illness.

IIIe: Experimental physicians
would report spending significantly more time with emotionally disturbed patients than did
control physicians.

As consultees learned that the emotionally disturbed individual needed much
reassurance and support and perhaps several
visits to the physician during the critical
stages of his illness, it was expected he
would report spending more time with the
person who had emotional problems.

POSSIBLE REINFORCERS OPERATING
TO CHANGE PHYSICIAN BEHAVIOR

Physicians who participated in the
first phase of the consultation program
mentioned that information provided by
the consultant regarding drugs, diagnosis,
treatment, history taking, referrals, and
the emotional support he provided them in
working with the mentally ill were very
valuable to them. It was believed that
these same characteristics might be

operating to bring about change in physician behavior during the second phase of
the program. One of the problems in determining whether reinforcement occurs in
social research is the difficulty in identifying what reinforcers, if any, are
operating to change behavior. It is possible that the following reinforcers were
operating to change physician behavior:

1.   information from a pres-
     tigious figure or expert,

2.   emotional support from the
     consultant in dealing with
     the emotionally disturbed
     patient,

3.   escape from an aversive
     situation of inability to
     deal with the emotionally
     disturbed patient, and

4.   job satisfaction on the
     part of the physician for
     dealing more effectively
     with the emotionally dis-
     turbed patient.

Information was obtained from the
interview schedule in order to determine
if these four reinforcers were operating
to change behavior.

Communication from a Prestigious Figure or Expert

Initially, the consultant may serve
as a reinforcer for the establishment of
new behaviors because the communications

he delivers might be seen as coming from
an expert or prestigious figure. Consultants have had special training in the
area of mental health, and it is possible
they were perceived as very knowledgeable
by the physicians. In our society, individuals who have a great deal of knowledge are generally seen as experts or pos-
sessors of a certain amount of prestige.
The studies on communicator credibility
demonstrate that attitude change occurs
more often and even in a direction discrepant from the subject's original position when the communicator has high credibility.

Emotional Support from the Consultant

The consultant may also be seen as
rewarding to the physician because he can
provide him emotional support in dealing
with the difficult problems the mental
patient presents. The very presence of
the consultant or his availability by
phone or visit when needed may be seen by
the physician as supportive. The consultant may often encourage the physician to
continue some of the same methods he is
currently using in treating the mental
patient, or he may inform him of a new
method and reward him verbally when he
uses a new type of treatment technique.

Escape from an Aversive Situation

It is possible that a physician might
feel uncomfortable working with emotionally

disturbed patients when he knows he does
not have the skills or knowledge to bring
them relief. The acquisition of new information that enables him to better understand the patient, and new information
about drugs or community resources that
helps the patient, might be seen as positive reinforcers by which he could escape
from an aversive situation of inability to
deal with the emotionally disturbed patient.

Job Satisfaction

After the consultant serves as a reinforcer for the initiation of new behavior, the new behaviors might be maintained
through the relationship the physician
develops with his patients. If the physician tries new behaviors and finds them to
be effective, he might experience an increase in job satisfaction. Job satisfaction would then serve as a reinforcer to
maintain the new behavior.

CHRONOLOGICAL DESCRIPTION OF EVENTS
THAT OCCURRED DURING
THE 1970-1972 PHASE OF THE PROGRAM

The major difference between the first
and second phases of the consultation program was that during the second phase the
goals of the program were identified prior
to the initiation of the program. During
the early months of 1971, one of the project directors (psychiatric consultant)
and the research psychologist met with the
seven consultants, individually and in

groups, to discuss the goals and evaluation
of the program. The following ideal goals
of the program were identified:

1. increase physician understanding and acceptance of
the emotionally disturbed
patient,

2. teach physicians how to
recognize the emotional
components of physical illness and understand that
emotional conflicts occur
with most any physical illness,

3. teach the physician the
importance of providing
local community care for
the patient where he can
receive support from family
and friends,

4. help physicians identify
those cases he can handle
himself and those that need
to be referred to another
resource,

5. provide physicians with
emotional support while
learning new treatment approaches,

6. inform physicians of local
community resources available to him and how to use
them most appropriately.

The consultants wanted to teach physicians about appropriate medications to use with the emotionally disturbed patient; how to deal with the individual with marital problems; and the depressed, alcoholic, geriatric, or adolescent patient.

The consultants provided the research psychologist with names of physicians who they thought would be interested in receiving consultation. Physicians were informed that the North Carolina Department of Mental Health had provided funds for consultants to help interested physicians with patients who had mental health problems. Some of the physicians had participated in an earlier phase of this project that was described in Chapter One. Physicians were randomly assigned to experimental and control groups after finding no significant differences between the groups on the variables of age, length of time in the community, medical specialty, urban or rural area, and previous number of consultation visits.

Since consultants agreed that one of their goals was to help physicians distinguish between the physical and emotional components of illness, the program co-director (psychiatric consultant) and research psychologist constructed a questionnaire designed to measure physician understanding of the psychiatric aspects of their patients' problems. Another goal was to increase physician understanding and acceptance of the mentally ill patient. We believed that an attitude scale which measured an increase in physician attitudes of social responsibility and a

decrease in attitudes of social distance
would give us some indication of the physicians' acceptance of the mentally ill patient. A group of psychiatrists who had
been in practice in North Carolina for at
least ten years was selected to help establish reliability of the instrument.
The first questionnaire was administered
to them in June 1971. During June 1971 additional meetings were held with the consultants to discuss the procedures for
administering the questionnaire to experimental and control physicians.

     Consultants contacted experimental and
control physicians either by phone or personal visit and asked them to complete the
questionnaires prior to the initiation of
consultation in June 1971. Control physicians were previously informed that they
would need to wait a year before receiving
consultation visits. Questionnaires were
either mailed to the consultee or delivered
to the consultee by the consultant. Consultants explained that all the responses
were confidential and would be seen only
by the research psychologist. The seven
consultants began consultation with the
experimental group after administration of
the pre-evaluation questionnaire. Consultants reported that few patient problems
were discussed the first month, June 1971,
because the consultant spent his time
explaining research procedures.

     The first consultation session in
which a patient was discussed was devoted
to building a relationship of trust with
the consultee. This was easier for consultants who lived in the physician's community because they were already known by

the physician and some trust may have been established through previous contacts. The consultants told the physicians the purpose of the consultation was to discuss any problems they were having with patients with emotional problems. Some of the physicians asked consultants to see certain patients whom they perceived as very difficult. This gave consultants an opportunity to demonstrate to the physician his skills in assessing the problem, making a diagnosis, arriving at a treatment plan, and using community resources. Two of the consultants saw patients for the physician although they told the physicians that they preferred to discuss the problem the physician was having with the patient rather than treat the patient. Consultants wanted physicians to become more confident of their own skills rather than relying upon the consultant to handle the problem. Their goal was not to teach physicians to become psychiatrists, but to build on the physicians' already existing strengths in working with the emotionally disturbed patient. As experimental physicians increased in understanding of the mentally ill patient and acquired additional skills in treating them, consultants reported that they saw fewer patients of the physician. Seeing or discussing patients who the physician thought were particularly difficult provided the consultant with an opportunity to identify content areas in which he should provide new information to the physician. The most frequent problems presented to the consultant were: (1) inability to distinguish physical illness from emotional illness, (2) lack of knowledge and skill in treating alcoholism and

depression, and (3) lack of information
about appropriate drugs for the emotionally disturbed patient. Consultants reported that they devoted entire sessions
to a discussion of these problem areas
and other resources in the community that
might help with these problems.

After consultants provided the physician with knowledge about problem cases,
an attempt was made to help the physician
recognize some of his own personal reactions to particular patients. Consultants
explained that it was only natural for
certain patients to create very negative
or positive feelings in physicians.

Several times during the evaluation
period, the co-director and research psychologist met with individual consultants
to discuss problems they were having in
conducting consultation. Consultants were
also asked to keep a progress record of
their consultation visits.

Problems during the Second Stage

After the new program had been in
effect for three months, several problems
occurred that forced us to examine the
feasibility of continuing the evaluation
of the program. During August 1971, three
consultants were dropped from the project
because expected state funds did not become available to continue the program in
two areas of the state, one consultant
moved out of the state, and the project
co-director (psychiatric consultant) re-
signed from the project. Only two of the

original consultants remained.

During the months of September, October, and most of November 1971, a decision for continuation of the project was pending. Continuation of the project was contingent upon hiring a new co-director (psychiatric consultant) and finding additional consultants. In mid-November 1971, a new co-director was employed, but he did not visit with physicians who were participating in the program as the previous two co-directors (psychiatric consultants) had done. Instead he was available to the consultants to discuss problems they were encountering during their consultation with the physicians in the program. After the new consultant joined the project in November 1971, a meeting was held with both co-directors, new consultants, the original two consultants, and the research psychologist to discuss long-range plans for the project. We decided to continue the project as originally designed, although the sample size was reduced, and to try to recruit at least one more consultant for the central area. In December 1971 consultation was resumed in the one county in the central area after the consultant was informed of the goals of the project, the research design, and the various phases of the project. The new consultant reported that he would try to continue consultation as it had been previously employed. A few weeks later a new consultant was hired for the second county in the central area of the state. The co-directors, the research psychologist, and one consultant who was familiar with the second county, discussed the history of the project and research

design with the second new consultant.
He stated that he intended to employ consultation as it was conducted by the previous consultant. At this time the sample
consisted of 21 experimental physicians
and 20 control physicians.

In January and February of 1972,
group meetings were conducted with all the
consultants to reassess goals and to share
information about the individual consultations. The consultant who was employed
in December died in February. After his
death no further consultation was performed in that county although efforts
were made to recruit another consultant.

During February 1972 the questionnaire was administered again to the original group of psychiatrists who completed
it in June of 1971. At the same time the
co-directors, consultants, and research
psychologist met to discuss administration
of the post-evaluation questionnaires at
the end of the evaluation period in June,
and to make arrangements for the research
psychologist to conduct personal interviews with each physician during July and
August of 1972.

In June 1972, postquestionnaires were
again mailed or delivered to the experimental and control physicians by the consultant. If a physician did not return
the questionnaire within a week or two, a
phone call was made to the physician ask-
ing him to please return the questionnaire
to the research psychologist.

Personal interviews were conducted
with all experimental and control

physicians during July and August of 1972.
Consultants had previously obtained permission for the interviews during their regular consultation visits with experimental
physicians and by phone from control physicians. Physicians were informed that
the research psychologist would interview
them in order to obtain their reactions
to consultation. A few weeks prior to the
interviews, consultants made definite ap-
pointments with the physicians by letter
and later confirmed them by phone calls
just prior to the scheduled interviews.
The research psychologist conducted 15- to
30-minute interviews with all 21 experimental and 19 of the 20 control physicians.
Only one control physician refused to participate. We believed we were successful
in obtaining information from the physicians because of the good relationship the
consultants had with the physicians, the
nominal sum they received for participating in the interviews, and the careful
planning and followup by the consultants
in scheduling and explaining the purpose
of the interviews.

    Consultation occurred in five areas
(thirteen counties) for three months from
June 1971 through August 1971. Because of
the problems previously described, consultation was employed in only three areas
(six counties) for ten months from June-
August 1971, and from December 1971-June
1972. One county in the third area received consultation for only five and one-
half months, from June-August 1971, and
December 1971 to mid-February 1972. Statistical analysis was conducted on all the
data from the three areas (seven counties)
where consultation was employed for ten

months and again including the data from
the one county where consultation was employed for only five and one-half months.
Since no significant differences were obtained between the two analyses, a decision was made to use the data from all
seven counties in three areas of the state.
No analyses were conducted in the areas
that received consultation for only three
months from June-August 1971.

The number of consultation visits
made to each physician was considered an
important part of the study, and each of
the participating group of physicians was
asked to give the number of visits they
had received from the consultant. Answers
ranged from none to twice a week by phone
or mail. Most consultees reported receiving an average of ten visits.

During progress meetings and again
at the end of the evaluation period in
June 1972, the research psychologist asked
consultants how many visits they made to
each consultee. All except one reported
they visited each consultee for approximately two hours once a month. One consultant reported that instead of visiting
each physician for two hours once a month
he visited his consultees during their
lunch hours for 30 minutes each week. The
average number of individual consultations
received by experimental physicians during
the time covered by the pre- and postadmin-
istration of the questionnaire was nine.

Consultants were paid for no more than
eight consultation days per month. It is
possible that some experimental physicians
may have received more or fewer visits

than the average of nine reported by the consultants and the average of ten reported by the consultees. Since this was not an evaluation of the role of the consultant, it was difficult for the research psychologist to obtain any more definite answer regarding number of visits other than the number reported by the physicians and by the consultants.

Evaluation of the second phase of the program ended in August 1972. The consultation program continued in three of the areas (six counties) through December 1973. A description of the program activities from August 1972 through December 1973 is reported in Appendix G.

REFERENCES

Aronson, E., Turner, J. A. & Carlsmith, J. M. Communicator credibility and communication discrepancy as determinants of opinion change. *Journal of Abnormal and Social Psychology*, 1963, *67*, 31-36.

Bergin, A. E. The effect of dissonant persuasive communications upon changes in a self-referring attitude. *Journal of Personality*, 1962, *30*, 423-428.

Bindman, A. J. The clinical psychologist as a mental health consultant. In L. E. Abt & B. F. Riess (Eds.) *Progress in clinical psychology*. New York: Grune and Stratton, 1966.

Caplan, G. *The theory and practice of mental health consultation*. New York: Basic Books, 1970.

Choo, T.   Communicator credibility and
    communication discrepancy as deter-
    minants of opinion change. *Journal
    of Social Psychology*, 1964, *64*, 65-76.
Cohen, A. R. *Attitude change and social in-
    fluence.*   New York: Basic Books,
    1964.
Ekman, P.   A comparison of verbal and
    non-verbal behavior as reinforcing
    stimuli of opinion responses.   Un-
    published doctoral dissertation,
    Adelphi College, Garden City, New
    York, 1958.
Greenspoon, J.   The reinforcing effect of
    two spoken words on the frequency of
    two responses. *American Journal of Psy-
    chology*, 1955, *68*, 409-416.
Hildum, D. C. & Brown, R. W.   Verbal re-
    inforcement and interviewer bias.
    Journal of Abnormal and Social Psychology,
    1956, *53*, 108-111.
Hovland, C. I. & Weiss, W.   The influence
    of source credibility on communica-
    tion effectiveness. *Public Opinion
    Quarterly*, 1951, *15*, 635-650.
Kelman, H. & Hovland, C. I.   "Reinstate-
    ment" of the communicator in delayed
    measurement of opinion change. *Jour-
    nal of Abnormal and Social Psychology*,
    1953, *48*, 327-335.
Krasner, L., Knowles, I. B. & Ullman,
    L. P.   Effect of verbal conditioning
    of attitudes on subsequent motor per-
    formance. *Journal of Personality and
    Social Psychology*, 1965, *1*, 407-412.
Lamson, W. C.   Personal Correspondence.
    National Institute of Mental Health,
    Rockville, Maryland, January, 1974.
Mannino, F. V. & Shore, M. F.   Consulta-
    tion research in mental health and
    related fields.   Public Health

Monograph No. 79, Public Health Service Publication No. 2122, U. S. Department of Health, Education, and Welfare, U. S. Government Printing Office, Washington, D. C., 1971.

Singer, R. D.   Verbal conditioning and generalization of pro-democratic responses. *Journal of Abnormal and Social Psychology*, 1961, *63*, 43-46.

Vacher, C. D.   Changes in knowledge, attitudes, and skills as a function of mental health consultation to physicians.   Unpublished doctoral dissertation, North Carolina State University, Raleigh, North Carolina, 1973.

Van Matre, R. M.   National institute of mental health and postgraduate education in psychiatry, In *Proceedings of the Third Colloquium for Postgraduate Teaching of Psychiatry*.   Washington, D. C.: American Psychiatric Association, 1964.

Zabarenko, L., Pittenger, R. A. & Zabarenko, R. N. *Primary Medical Practice*. St. Louis, Missouri: Warren H. Green, 1968.

3. METHOD

Since instruments measuring the goals
we wished to implement were not available,
we developed our own case vignettes and
interview schedule. The social responsibility and social distance scale had been
used previously with several groups to
measure mental health attitudes, but not
with a physician population. We believed
that the social distance and social responsibility scale would provide us with
an accurate measure of attitude change if
it was validated on a criterion group of
physicians.

SAMPLE

Seven consultants residing in five
different areas of the state of North Carolina provided lists of physicians who they
thought would be interested or who had expressed interest in receiving psychiatric
consultation. This procedure resulted in
an original sample of 80 physicians. Forty

physicians were randomly assigned to the experimental group and forty to the control group within the constraints that the two groups were balanced with regard to factors of residence (rural or urban area) and type of practice (general practice, obstetrics, gynecology, surgery, pediatrics). A Mann Whitney U test indicated the two groups were similar in age, length of time in the community, and number of previous consultation visits. In order to establish the experimental and control groups and still maintain the interest of participants, the experimental group of physicians was told it would receive psychiatric consultation during the first year of the program while the control physicians were told they would receive consultation the second year. Because of the modifications in the original program that were described in an earlier chapter, it was necessary to reduce the sample to 20 control and 21 experimental physicians. Questionnaires were returned by only 10 control and 15 experimental physicians. Interview information was obtained from 19 control and 21 experimental physicians. Physicians were more responsive to the interviews because personal visits were made to physicians and they were paid for participating in each interview.

DESCRIPTION OF INSTRUMENTS
USED IN COLLECTING DATA

Case Studies

Since one of the goals of the

consultation program was to teach physicians how to recognize the emotional components of physical illness and learn how to refer the emotionally disturbed patient to appropriate resources, an instrument measuring this type of knowledge was needed in order to determine if the consultation program was effective in changing this aspect of physician behavior. We believed that case studies which gave some information about emotional factors often involved in mental illness, and just enough information to merit the possibility of an organic illness, could provide a measure of physician achievement about mental illness. Physicians were first asked to identify etiology, diagnostic approach, clinical impression, treatment plan, and appropriate referral resource for the individual described in each case study. Next, they were asked to rank four options under each of the above five categories. Verification of the case studies is discussed in Appendix F. After the case study item reliabilities were established, a "standard score" or "judges" score was then computed. First, the seven pre- and post-responses to each of the items were summed. Dividing by the number of observations gave an average of each of these which yielded a single rank for each of the four options to the 14 questions.

Once the ranks were established, differences between a standard validating rank score and each experimental or control rank was obtained for the four options within each of the 14 questions. The scores for a single item, j, for a single subject, i, were obtained as follows: Physician A's response to option one (VI) was subtracted from that of the average validating rank for option one (01) and then squared. Options two, three, and four (02, 03, 04) were treated the same. The squared differences for the four options were summed to obtain a score for each of the 14 identified reliable items.

The case studies were selected as a measure of physician knowledge of emotional illness because Pearson & Lee (1969) had reported they were useful. They used the case studies to measure the cognitive knowledge of physicians who participated in seminars on the emotional aspects of physical illness. Taylor (1961) also found case studies useful in distinguishing treatment patterns for emotionally disturbed patients among a group of general practitioners and a group of psychiatrists. In a study conducted by Rozan & Holmes (1968), they recommended that an appropriate instrument for physician evaluation might be one which could determine decision-making regarding diagnosis, treatment, and referral.

Social Distance and Social Responsibility Scale

The social distance and social responsibility attitude scale was used as another measure of the effectiveness of the consultation program in changing physician behavior. We believed that as physicians became more informed about mental health and mental illness and new or alternate ways of treating the emotionally disturbed patient, they would increase in understanding of the mentally ill person.

As they became more understanding of the
mentally ill person, it was believed they
would acquire more accepting attitudes
toward him which would be reflected in an
increase in attitudes of social responsibility and a decrease in attitudes of
social distance toward the mentally ill.
A fifteen-item social distance and social
responsibility scale was chosen to measure
these attitudes.

Physicians were asked to rate their
feelings with regard to the 15 social
distance and social responsibility statements. Answers to these statements were
to be made on a one to five scale which
indicated a range of feeling from strong
agreement to strong disagreement. Theo-
retically, scores could range from a low
of 15, indicating a strong agreement response to an item, to 75, indicating a
strong disagreement response to each item
in the scale. Responses to the negatively
worded items three, 11, and 13 were scored
oppositely to direction implied by response prior to the summing of item responses to give a total score.

The social distance and social responsibility scale used in the present
study was first used by Cumming & Cumming
(1957) to measure mental health attitudes
of a conservative Canadian community
toward a mental health education program.
Social distance was defined by Cumming &
Cumming (1957) as the degree of relationship the respondent is willing to tolerate
with someone who has been mentally ill.
Social responsibility referred to a person's feelings of responsibility for
causing illness as well as feelings of

responsibility for assuming the social
burden which the mentally ill person places
on society.

Social distance items were also used
by Edgerton & Bentz (1969) in their assessment of the attitudes of rural people
toward the mentally ill. Positive responses ranged from 87.79 per cent (they
would be willing to work with someone who
had been mentally ill) to 43.90 per cent
(they could conceive of themselves falling
in love with a mentally ill person).

Another study showed the scales to
differentiate between groups. Bentz et al
(1970) used six social distance items and
five social responsibility items to compare the attitudes of a highly rural and
stable population with a group of high
school teachers. Surprisingly, teachers
who were better educated than the general
public showed more attitudes of social
distance and fewer social responsibility
attitudes toward the mentally ill.

Five of these social distance items
were used by Phillips in several studies
involving the same sample to determine
social distance to social and demographic
variables. In the first study (1963),
five social distance items were used to
measure degree of rejection of the mentally
ill person. The social distance items
were similar, but worded differently from
those used in the previously mentioned
studies. Three hundred married white
females living in a small New England town
were presented with five cards which described behavior (of a paranoid schizophrenic, a simple schizophrenic, an

anxious-depressed person) and help-source utilized (no help, clergyman, physician, psychiatrist, and mental hospital). Using the social distance items as a rejection score, it was found that individuals who saw a psychiatrist or used the mental hospital were most rejected.

In the second study, Phillips (1964) presented subjects with the five descriptions of behavior, but this time the actor was presented as male in one half of the situations and as female in the other half. After the subjects were presented with the abstracts and help-source utilized, the social distance items were used to measure how close a relationship the subjects were able to tolerate with the characters in the question situations. Phillips found that males were rejected more strongly than females and rejection was based on how visibly the behavior deviated from customary role expectations rather than the pathology of the behavior.

The third study was conceived to determine the willingness of subjects to associate with individuals as described in the abstracts and again when the individuals in the abstracts were reported to have been in a mental hospital (Phillips, 1966). Almost three-fourths of the subjects reported they would be willing to have the paranoid schizophrenic for a neighbor, but fewer than two per cent would allow their children to marry someone so described. When the individuals were described as having been hospitalized, rejection increased. Only 17 per cent of the respondents would allow their children to marry a normal individual if he had once been in a mental hospital.

Crocetti & Lemkau (1963) conducted
a survey of low-income residents in Balti-
more as a preliminary step in a study of
the feasibility of community based psychiatric emergency and home care programs.
They were interested in trying to understand popular feeling about psychiatric
home care programs and thought information
on how seriously the public regards mental
illness as compared to other illnesses was
important. They used 11 items measuring
attitudes toward mental illness. The
items constituted what the authors called
enlightened or unenlightened attitudes
toward the mentally ill. Four of these
items were the same social responsibility
and social distance items used in the
present study, while the other seven were
similar but worded differently. No score
was obtained and only percentages reported.

In another study Crocetti et al (1971)
used two questions about mental illness
and three social distance items to measure
attitudes toward the mentally ill in a
blue collar population. A weighted index
of social distance was obtained by com-
bining both the degree of social distance
and the intensity of feeling ranging over
five categories from definitely willing
to definitely unwilling. Using the three
social distance items they found that
almost fifteen times as many people gave
totally accepting responses as gave totally rejecting ones. They concluded that
there was no evidence of extreme rejection
of the mentally ill by blue collar workers.

Several studies have used the social

distance and social responsibility scales
but the same items were not always used,
the wording of some of the items was
changed, and results were sometimes reported as percentages rather than scores.
Because of these inconsistencies it was
necessary to establish reliability of the
15 items used in the present study with
a group of psychiatrists before administering them to the experimental and control physicians.

*Referrals to Mental Hospitals and Mental Health
Centers*

In order to determine if the consultation program had changed performance
skills of physicians, information on the
number and type of referrals to mental
hospitals and mental health centers was
obtained. It was first necessary to identify which physicians were making referrals to the mental hospitals. Names of
patients referred to the three mental
hospitals in the three geographical areas
covered by the project were obtained from
the Statistics Division of the North Carolina Department of Mental Health. In
North Carolina individuals who need to be
admitted to a mental hospital are assigned
to the mental hospital in their geographic
area. For example, patients of physicians
in the New Hanover area are admitted to
Cherry Hospital, patients in Lee and Harnett Counties to Dorothea Dix Hospital,
and patients in the New River Mental
Health Center area to Broughton Hospital
(see map, Appendix A).

After all patients admitted to these three hospitals for the periods January-June 1971 and January-June 1972 were identified, only those referred by experimental or control physicians were counted. Number and type of referrals were recorded for each experimental and control physician.

Data on the number and type of referrals to the mental health centers were obtained from (the New Hanover, New River, Lee and Harnett Mental Health Centers) mental health centers in each of the three project areas of the state. Information was obtained by pulling all patient folders for 1971 and 1972 and selecting only those seen by experimental and control physicians for the periods January-June 1971 and January-June 1972. After experimental and control physicians making the referrals were identified, number and type of referral were recorded for each. The total number of psychiatric referrals and the total number of alcoholic and geriatric referrals to mental health centers and mental hospitals was obtained for each experimental and control physician.

Interview Schedule

The interview schedule (see Appendix D) was designed by the research psychologist to obtain information about physician attitudes and performance skills. Several questions were asked in more than one format in order to insure that the desired information was obtained. Questions were asked concerning (1) referrals to community agencies, (2) use of community

resources, (3) discussion of patients with
emotional problems with others, (4) drug
prescription patterns, (5) amount of time
spent with psychiatric patients, (6) comfort in working with psychiatric patients,
(7) perception of the medical certification process, and (8) view of others.
Other questions were asked (see Appendix
D), but were not included in the analysis
because the researcher either believed
the question was poor, misunderstood by
the physician, or physicians stated they
were not able to give a valid response to
the item.

INSTRUMENT VERIFICATION

In order to establish reliability of
the instruments the questionnaire contain-
ing the case studies and social distance
and social responsibility scale was administered to a group of psychiatrists in
North Carolina who had been in practice
for at least ten years. During May 1971,
15 psychiatrists were sent letters inviting
them to participate in the study. Thirteen psychiatrists returned the questionnaires. These same psychiatrists were
asked to complete the questionnaire for
the second time in February 1972. Nine
complete pairs of questionnaires were
used in the final analysis.

Analysis of variance techniques were
used to establish reliability of the case
studies and the social distance and social
responsibility scale. These procedures
are discussed in Appendix F.

SUMMARY

The case studies and interview schedule were developed and validated for use
with a physician population. These same
instruments could be modified to measure
knowledge, attitudes, and skills of nurses,
teachers, lawyers, ministers, or other
community groups who may participate in a
mental health consultation program.

REFERENCES

Bentz, W. K., Hollister, W. G. & Kherlo-
    pian, M. Attitudes of social dis-
    tance and responsibility for mental
    illness: a comparison of teachers
    and the general public. *Psychology in
    the Schools*, 1970, *7* (2),198-203.
Crocetti, G. M. & Lemkau, P. V. Public
    opinion of psychiatric home care in
    an urban area. *American Journal of Public
    Health*, 1963, *53*,409-414.
Crocetti, G., Spiro, H. L. & Siassi, I.
    Are the ranks closed? Attitudinal
    social distance and mental illness.
    American Journal of Psychiatry, 1971, *127*
    (9),1121-1127.
Cumming, E. & Cumming, J. *Closed ranks: an
    experiment in mental health education.*   Cam-
    bridge, Massachusetts: Harvard Uni-
    versity Press, 1957.
Edgerton, J. W. & Bentz, W. K. Attitudes
    and opinions of rural people about
    mental illness and program services.
    American Journal of Public Health, 1969,
    59 (3),470-477.

Pearson, J. B. & Lee, A.   Questionnaire analysis of three seminars, 1967-1968.   In J. B. Pearson (Ed.) *The assessment of short-term seminars in psychiatry for non-psychiatrist physicians: a progress report for the years 1966-68.* Boulder, Colorado: Western Interstate Commission for Higher Education, 1969.

Phillips, D. L.   Rejection: a possible consequence of seeking help for mental disorders. *American Sociological Review,* 1963, *28,*963-972.

Phillips, D. L.   Rejection of the mentally ill: the influence of behavior and sex. *American Sociological Review,* 1964, *29,* 679-687.

Phillips, D. L.   Public identification and acceptance of the mentally ill. *American Journal of Public Health,* 1966, *56,* 755-763.

Rozan, G. H. & Holmes, D.   Evaluating the impact of a psychiatric course for non-psychiatric physicians. *Mental Hygiene,* 1968, *52,*612-616.

Taylor, J. B.   The psychiatrist and the general practitioner. *Archives of general psychiatry,* 1961, *5,*1-6.

4. RESULTS OF THE SECOND PHASE OF THE PROGRAM

The results of the evaluation conducted during the second phase of the consultation program are presented in the following four sections. Whenever possible, comparisons are made on information obtained during the first and second phases of the project. Part one presents results of the case studies which measure physician knowledge about etiology, diagnostic approach, clinical impression, treatment approach, and referral resource for the emotionally disturbed patient. In part two information on the attitudes of physicians toward the mentally ill is presented. This includes the attitudinal measures of social distance and social responsibility and interview responses about perceptions of the medical certification process, view of others, and comfort in working with psychiatric patients. Performance skills of physicians are discussed in part three. This includes information on drug prescription patterns, referrals to mental hospitals and mental health centers, discussion of patients with emotional problems with others, use of community resources, and time spent with psychiatric patients. In order to support some of the theoretical considerations of the study, procedural check information concerning information about perceptions of the consultant's knowledge, emotional support from the consultant, confidence in working with the emotionally disturbed patient, and job satisfaction is presented.

I.   RESULTS OF THE ACHIEVEMENT MEASURES OF PHYSICIAN KNOWLEDGE

One of the major hypotheses of the study was that physicians would increase in their knowledge of mental health and their ability to deal effectively with the mentally ill person. The case studies were chosen as an instrument to measure increase in knowledge of experimental physicians regarding etiology, clinical impression, diagnostic approach, treatment, and referral resource for the emotionally disturbed patient. The experimental and control groups were believed to be equivalent in knowledge about mental health and mental illness prior to initiation of consultation because of the selection procedures that were discussed in an earlier chapter. It was expected they would obtain similar pretest scores on the case studies. An inspection of means (Table 1) shows the two groups were similar in their knowledge of psychiatric approaches to mental illness as reflected in scores on the case study questions.

Table 1
Means and Standard Deviations for Experimental and Control Groups on Case Studies

	Experimental (N=15)		Control (N=10)	
	Mean	S.D.	Mean	S. D.
Pre	50.65	18.52	49.59	19.36
Post	56.61	17.01	49.18	16.72

Results of an analysis of variance on the pretest showed no significant differences (F<1) between the experimental and control groups. We concluded the two groups were equivalent in their knowledge of mental health concepts and effectiveness in dealing with the mental health problems presented in the case studies at the time consultation began.

As the experimental group learned more about mental health concepts during the consultation sessions, it was hypothesized they would move closer to the validating group on the post-test. Only the experimental group was expected to show an improvement (lower score) from pre- to post-tests. Lack of differences (F, N.S.) between the two groups on the post-test did not support the expectation that the experimental group would move toward the more approved rankings of the validating group of psychiatrists.

We concluded that consultation had no effect on the experimental physicians as measured by the case studies. The consultant's original goal was to teach physicians about medication, depression, alcoholic, geriatric, and marital problems

during their visits. It is possible that
consultants did not have sufficient time
to provide physicians with a great deal
of information on the emotional components
of physical illness, and physicians may
have needed additional consultation sessions in order to learn the specifics of
etiology, clinical impression, diagnostic
approach, treatment, and referral for the
emotionally disturbed patient. As was
mentioned earlier, several changes occurred in the project; loss of the director and consultants, and a two and one-
half month interruption of the project
before other consultants and co-directors
were employed. Enelow & Adler (1964),
Pearson & Young (1966), and Zabarenko et
al (1968), who evaluated the psychiatric
skills of general practitioners, stated
that few changes can be observed in a
period of time as short as a year. Other
studies have reported that learning occurred among physicians when participation
was longer than one year. For example,
Pittenger (1962) found that out of 30
physicians who participated in his seminars over a three-year period, 27 reported
they understood patients better and 24
stated they had better recognition of emotional problems. Forman et al (1964)
observed no change in the knowledge of
physicians who participated in his psychiatric seminars for only one year, but
after the second year these same physicians were in agreement with a criterion
group of psychiatrists in understanding
the personalities of their patients, and
in recognition of the importance of attitudes and personalities of doctors. A
similar finding was reported by Enelow
(1966) and Enelow & Adler (1964). Six

physicians who participated in the program for more than one year showed a
marked improvement in their ability to
evaluate psychiatric disturbances. Interviews with these six students indicated that the greater the amount of participation in the program, the greater
the ability to evaluate psychiatric disturbances.

The above mentioned studies found
that length of participation in a psychiatric education program produced the
greatest amount of attitude change in
physicians, but Dorsey et al (1964) observed that frequency of contact within
a shorter period of time may be just as
effective. Dorsey et al observed changes
in knowledge and attitudes of public
health nurses during a five-month period
after participating in weekly conferences
conducted by psychiatrists, psychiatric
social workers, and mental health nurses
who were also available as consultants
during the week. The greatest change occurred in nursing knowledge, nursing practices, and attitudes toward patients.
Nurses increased in their understanding
of individual and family psychodynamics,
and their understandings were more like
the consultants at the end of the five-
month program.

These studies indicate that length
of time in the program or frequency of
contact with the consultant appear to be
related to the amount of learning that
occurs in the consultee group.

II.   RESULTS OF MEASURES OF ATTITUDE

A second major hypothesis of the study was that physician attitudes toward mental health or the mentally ill would become more positive after participating in the consultation program. Results of the social distance and social responsibility measures of attitudes are presented in this section. Other attitudinal measures obtained from personal interviews with the physicians are also reported. These include physician perceptions of the medical certification process, comfort in working with emotionally disturbed patients, confidence in working with psychiatric patients, and view of others. A description of the hypotheses, analysis procedures, and results are presented separately for each of the measures.

A. *Social Distance and Social Responsibility Scale*

In order to determine if consultation had influenced physician attitudes toward the mentally ill, it was hypothesized that experimental physician scores on the post-questionnaire would be significantly lower than the scores of control group physicians. One of the assumptions that needed to be tested before the hypothesis could be considered was that experimental and control groups would show no significant differences in their total presocial distance and social responsibility scale scores.

In Table 2, an inspection of means for the two administrations shows little

Table 2
Means and Standard Deviations
for Experimental and Control Groups
on Pre- and Postattitude Scales

	Experimental (N=15)		Control (N=10)	
	Mean	S.D.	Mean	S.D.
Pre	35.40	5.82	36.30	7.12
Post	36.93	5.97	36.70	6.16

change for either group. Results of an
analysis of variance (F<1) (experimental
versus control) showed there were no significant differences between the two
groups on the social distance and social
responsibility scale scores prior to consultation.

Since no reliable differences on the
pretest measures were obtained, it was
assumed that differences as a result of
the treatment would be obtained from the
derived postprogram attitude scale scores.
An analysis of variance technique (F<1)
again indicated no significant differences
on social distance and social responsibility attitudes between the group which
received the consultation and the group
which did not have access to this service.
Therefore, we concluded there was no support for the contention that physician
attitudes toward the mentally ill would
change as a function of consultation with
experts. Most of the items in the social
distance and social responsibility scale
measured attitudes toward the severely
disturbed patient or persons who required
hospitalization. It is possible that physicians may have changed their attitudes

toward the mildly disturbed individual although the instrument did not measure these attitudes.

B. *Perception of the Medical Certification Process*

It was hypothesized that experimental physicians would find the medical certification process less cumbersome after participating in the consultation program. Since physicians in general have been dissatisfied with the time consuming procedures for committing patients to mental hospitals, it was believed that both experimental and control physicians would be in agreement on this question prior to consultation. Results of the chi square analysis (Table 3) showed the experimental group perceived the medical certification process as less difficult (x^2=6.44, df=3, p<.10) after consultation.

This indicates that the experimental group learned about the procedures necessary for committing patients to the mental hospital from their participation in the consultation program. This finding is consistent with information obtained from physicians who participated in the 1964-1967 phase of the project in the western part of the state. These physicians also reported that the consultant had been helpful to them in learning the necessary procedures for commitment to the mental hospital.

Table 3

Physician Perception of the Medical Certification Process

Difficulty in Medical Certification to Mental Hospital	Experimental		Control	
	Frequency	Per cent	Frequency	Per cent
Yes	7	35	5	28
No	13	65	8	44
No Change	0	0	5	28
Omits	1	0	1	0
	21	100	18	100

C.   Physicians' Views of Others

It was believed that experimental physicians would report that they viewed nurses, office workers, physicians, and others with whom they worked with increased sensitivity after their knowledge of mental health concepts increased. Since it was predicted that physicians would increase in social responsibility and social distance toward the mentally ill, it was assumed that they would become more accepting of the behavior of others. We also believed that physicians would acquire more accepting attitudes toward others from observing the consultant's behavior. As can be noted from Table 4, the hypothesis was supported, (x^2=4.04, df=1, p<.05). These results are consistent with conclusions reached in other studies measuring the effectiveness of consultation. A study by Schmuck (1968) reported that teachers who received consultation from psychiatrists, psychologists, and social workers changed their self perceptions and improved their views on how to handle classroom problems. Caplan (1970) found that public health nurses improved in professional objectivity after three years of mental health consultation, and Norman & Forti (1972) also reported that consultees from thirteen community agencies believed that consultation from nurses, social workers, and psychologists was helpful in broadening their view of problems and in providing objective views of a situation.

Table 4
Physicians' Views of Other People

Change	Experimental		Control	
	Frequency	Per cent	Frequency	Per cent
Yes	8	38.1	2	10.5
No	13	61.9	17	89.4
	21	100.0	19	99.9

91

D. Comfort in Working with Patients

As experimental physicians worked
with the consultants and gained more understanding of the emotionally disturbed
patient and how to care for him, it was
expected they would report a change in
the type of patients with whom they felt
more comfortable. The summarized responses are given in Table 5. Twenty-
five per cent of the experimental and
twelve per cent of the controls reported
they felt more comfortable in working with
certain patients. However, this difference was not significant ($x^2=1.37$, df=1,
p>.10).

This finding was unexpected since a
previous study had reported that physicians who participated in their seminars
gained insight into their own problems
which in turn helped reduce tensions in
working with others who had similar problems (Brody et al, 1965). Another study
by Pittenger (1962) found that physicians
had less anxiety about patients who had
emotional problems after the course was
over, and Greco (1966), a general practitioner, reported a decreased fear in lis-
tening for the underlying emotional problem after participating in psychiatric
seminars for one and one-half years.

III.   RESULTS OF CHANGE IN PERFOR-
       MANCE SKILLS OF PHYSICIANS

The following section presents the
results of information obtained about phy-

Table 5

Perceived Change in Comfort in Working
with Emotionally Disturbed Patients

	Experimental		Control	
	Frequency	Per cent	Frequency	Per cent
Change	5	.25	2	.11
No Change	15	.75	17	.89
	20	100.00	19	100.00

93

sician drug prescription patterns and
referrals to mental hospitals and mental
health centers. These are observable behaviors which show change in physicians
from one year to the next and indicate
the effectiveness of consultation. Referral information which is reported in part
one was obtained from the Statistics Division of the North Carolina Department of
Mental Health and the mental health centers in each physician's geographical
area. Drug information, reported in part
two, was obtained from the personal interviews conducted with each physician. Additional measures of change were also
obtained from the interviews and these
results are presented in the last four
parts of the chapter. Measures of change
in performance skills include physician
use of community resources, discussion of
patient problems with others, time spent
with psychiatric patients, and patients
requiring the most time.

A.   *Drug Prescription Patterns*

Since part of the consultation program involved educating physicians about
the use of drugs for the emotionally disturbed patient, we thought the experimental group would be significantly different
from the controls in prescribing drugs for
the psychiatric patient.

As experimental physicians learned
more about drugs, it was expected they

would prescribe more major tranquilizers*
and antidepressants[+] for the severely disturbed psychiatric patient. It was also
thought that the experimental physicians
would prescribe fewer barbiturates[o] and
more major and minor tranquilizers[Δ] for
the mildly disturbed patient and nonpsychiatric patient in a crisis situation.
Results of the categorical data analysis
provided support for these hypotheses.
Experimental physicians prescribed major
tranquilizers and antidepressants for
severely disturbed patients more often
than control physicians (x^2=3.7176, df=1,
p<.10). The experimental group also prescribed more tranquilizers (both major and
minor) and fewer barbiturates for the
mildly disturbed patient than did the control group (x^2=4.055, df=1, p<.05). However, no such pattern could be discerned
for the experimental and control physicians when handling nonpsychotic patients
in crisis situations (x^2=.09, df=1, p>.10).

These findings regarding drug prescription patterns are important because

---

*Major tranquilizers are psychotropic
 drugs used primarily for alleviating
 symptoms of psychotic disorder; for example, the phenothiazines.
[+]Antidepressants are major tranquilizers
 that have mood elevating effects for persons with depressive symptoms; for example, the tricyclicamines.
[o]Barbiturates are sedatives of differing
 varieties of barbituric acid--the primary
 effect is sedation.
[Δ]Minor tranquilizers are drugs that are
 used primarily to reduce anxiety.

Table 6
Drug Prescription Patterns

	Severely Disturbed		Mildly Disturbed		Nonpsychiatric Patient in Crisis Situation	
	E	C	E	C	E	C
Major Tranquilizers	34	19	13	6	1	0
Antidepressants	10	5	21	14	4	3
Minor Tranquilizers	4	18	13	31	26	29
Barbiturates	0	0	2	11	7	9
Total Number of Responses	48	42	49	62	38	41

Table 7
Influence on Drug Prescription Patterns

	Experimental		Control	
Categories	Rankings	Weighted Totals	Rankings	Weighted Totals
Consultants	1	55	2	42
Journals	2	42	1	49
Other Physicians	3	36		
Pharmaceutical Representatives	4	16	3	26
Experience	5	14	4	16

proper medication can ameliorate unwanted
symptoms and help maintain individuals in
their home communities. The fact that
fewer barbiturates were prescribed for
mentally disturbed patients by experimental physicians has important implications
for the drug problem currently facing our
society. Physicians who prescribe tranquilizers rather than barbiturates may be
able to play a small role in preventing
increased depression in the currently depressed individual and prevent other individuals from becoming habitual barbiturate
users.

An assumption of the study was that
experimental physicians would perceive the
consultant as more influential in changing
their drug prescription patterns than
journals, pharmaceutical representatives,
or other physicians. (Some physicians
gave sources other than the four previously named, e.g., experience). A weighted
total for each category was derived where-
by the source considered most important
would be assigned a "4," the next most important, a "3," the next, a "2," and the
least important, a "1." It should be
noted that physicians ranked as few as one
and as many as four of the categories.
The scores were then added up for each
source of information to provide the rankings listed below. As Table 7 illustrates,
the experimental group ranked consultants
highest.

When the consultants category was
dropped from consideration, the experimental and control group differed only
on the ranking of the first two catego-

ries. The experimental group believed
journals were more helpful after consultation, while the control group believed
it was influenced most by other physicians. Pharmaceutical representatives
and experience were ranked relatively low
by both groups. It is possible the experience category may have been perceived
as an important factor by physicians but
did not show up as a significant source,
since it was not one of the options presented by the interviewer. However, eight
physicians reported they considered this
factor to be most important.

Since the experimental group of physicians ranked the consultants as being
most influential in changing their drug
prescription patterns, we concluded that
the consultation program was effective
in changing experimental physicians' drug
prescription patterns. Physicians who
participated in the project from 1964-
1967 also reported that the consultant's
advice regarding medication was helpful.

B. *Referrals to Mental Hospitals and Mental
Health Centers*

Another hypothesis stated that experimental physicians would refer fewer
patients to mental hospitals and more to
mental health centers after participating
in the consultation program. If the experimental and control physicians were
comparable, then it seemed reasonable to
expect that the two groups would refer

the same number and type of patients to
the mental hospitals and mental health
centers in 1971. If the experimental physicians were learning to deal with the
emotionally disturbed patient through consultation, it was believed they would refer fewer patients to mental hospitals,
especially alcoholic and geriatric types,
and more to the mental health centers in
1972. The consultants believed they could
teach the consultees how to deal effectively with the alcoholic and geriatric
patient in the community. Table 8 presents the number of referrals to mental
hospitals and mental health centers by
year and by physician group. Since the
frequency of referrals was available on
a county basis for the physicians participating in the program, we decided to
use the county as the unit of analysis.
The ratio of the number of referrals to
the number of physicians was determined
separately for the control group and experimental group of physicians within each
county. Since a substantial amount of
variability existed between counties, it
was decided to perform a square root trans-
formation of the ratios in order to reduce
the variability in the data.

To ascertain the validity of the expectations of the researcher, an analysis
of variance was conducted on the transformed ratios which allowed the estimation
of effects due to factors in a year by
type of referral within the physician
group design. Since change in referral
patterns was expected from one year to the
next for the experimental physicians only,
this would represent an interaction of the

Table 8

Referrals to Mental Hospitals and Mental
Health Centers by Year and Group

	1971			1972		
	MH	MHC	Total	MH	MHC	Total
Experimental	107	60	167	76	57	133
Control	60	40	100	69	24	96
Total	167	100	267	145	84	229

factors of group, year, and type of referral (i.e., referral to mental health center or mental hospital). The three way
group by type of referral by year interaction was the only significant effect observed ($F=4.85$; $df=1$, 6; $p<.05$). Thus,
there was support for the researcher's
expectations. To assist in the interpre-
tation of the interaction, the ratio of
referrals by physicians per county were
plotted in Figure 1. As can be noted by
an inspection of the figure, only part of
the expected effect due to the experimental treatment took place. While the referrals made to mental hospitals by the
experimental physicians were fewer in 1972
than in 1971, their referrals to the local
mental health centers did not show the
expected increase. Also, the physicians
in the control group showed an unexpected
decrease in the usage of the community
mental health centers from 1971 to 1972
although their number of referrals to the
mental hospitals was the same.

We concluded that the consultation
program was effective in changing physician referral patterns to mental hospitals. It is believed they learned about
the importance of keeping the emotionally
disturbed patient in his home community.
This finding is consistent with a finding
from an earlier phase of the project in
which a decrease in admissions and readmissions to the state hospitals was observed in the project areas where consultation was employed.

However, it cannot be concluded that
the consultation program was influential

Figure 1*
Graph on Significant Iteration of Group
by Time by Year for Total Number of Referrals
to Mental Hospitals and Mental Health Centers

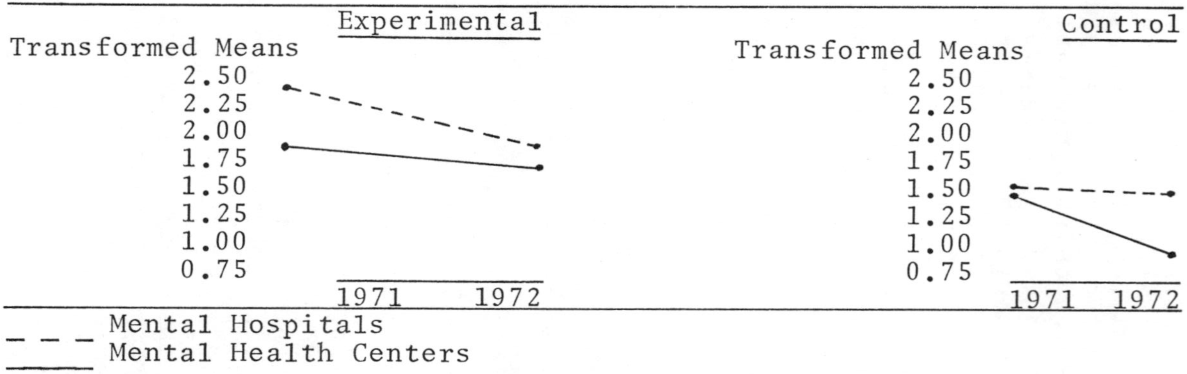

*The untransformed means were used because it was thought they would be easier to interpret.

in changing physician referral patterns
to the mental health centers, since the
experimental group did not increase in
total number of referrals as predicted.
A possible explanation for this may be
that experimental physicians became more
confident in treating the emotionally disturbed patient in their offices and did
not need to refer as many to the mental
health center. A similar view was reported by Pearson & Lee (1969) in their
attempt to change physician behavior
through participation in seminars. They
believed that referrals may not have increased because the consultees were accepting more responsibility in working
with emotionally disturbed patients.
Stephenson (1973) also found that a family
and welfare agency reported a decrease in
referrals to outside agencies after receiving mental health consultation for
three years.

The referral by year by group within
county analysis model was also used for
testing the expectation of the researchers
with regard to data on alcoholic referrals. The frequencies of alcoholic referrals to mental hospitals and mental
health centers by year and group are presented in Table 9.

The statistical analysis procedure
was performed on the same type of trans-
formation as used in the previous analysis.
That is, the square root of the ratio of
number of referrals to the number of physicians in the county served as the dependent variable. The results of the analysis of variance showed a highly significant referral effect ($F=44.4$, $df=1$, 6;

Table 9

Alcoholic Referrals to Mental Hospitals and
Mental Health Centers by Year and Group

	1971			1972		
	MH	MHC	Total	MH	MHC	Total
Experimental	79	9	88	69	3	72
Control	38	6	44	42	4	46
Total	117	15	132	111	7	118

Table 10

Geriatric Referrals to Mental Hospitals and
Mental Health Centers by Year and Group

	1971			1972		
	MH	MHC	Total	MH	MHC	Total
Experimental	3	3	6	10	3	13
Control	3	1	4	6	0	6
Total	6	4	10	16	3	19

104

p<.01) to be the only statistical reliable
outcome. As can be noted by an inspection
of Table 9, both experimental and control
group physicians made a substantially
greater number of referrals to the mental
hospitals as compared to the community
mental health centers. Physicians, on the
average, referred nine times as many patients to mental hospitals as to community
mental health centers for treatment of
alcoholism.

We concluded that the consultation
program had no effect on the number of
alcoholic patients referred to mental hospitals or mental health centers. It was
believed that experimental physicians as
they increased in understanding of the
alcoholic and alternative treatments for
him would either prefer to treat him in
their offices or refer him to the mental
health center. This finding is surprising
since physicians had mentioned alcoholic
patients as one of their major problems.

It was also expected that experimental physicians would decrease in the number of geriatric referrals made over time
to the mental hospital and increase in the
number of geriatric referrals to the mental health centers. The number of geriatric referrals by experimental and control
physicians to mental hospitals and mental
health centers for the years 1971 and 1972
is presented in Table 10.

Utilizing the same analysis procedures as conducted for the total number of
referrals and the number of alcoholic referrals, no statistically significant effects were found to account for the vari-

ance observed in the geriatric referrals
made by physicians in the study. Our expectations of change in physician behavior
with regard to geriatric patient referral
were not supported by the available data.

We concluded that the consultation
program was not effective in teaching physicians about the importance of maintaining the elderly patient in the community.
It is interesting to note that the total
number of patients over 65 who were referred to mental hospitals and mental
health centers was only ten for 1971 and
19 for 1972. These small totals might
indicate that these individuals were being
maintained in their home communities.

C. *Community Resources*

It was hypothesized that experimental
physicians would refer more patients to
community agencies as they learned of the
services they could provide to their patients and how to refer patients to them.
Low, median, and high levels of referrals
are reported in Table 11 by physicians
using these resources. This material
shows that the greatest number of referrals was made to the public health department by both experimental and control physicians. Experimental physicians ranked
using private psychiatrists most often
and the public health department and mental health center second most often. The
control group used the public health department most often, private psychiatrists
second, the welfare department third,

Table 11
Use of Community Resources

Resources	Experimental					Control					x^2
	N	Low	Median	High	Per cent Used	N	Low	Median	High	Per cent Used	
Public Health Department	21	0	25	>999	95.2	19	3	60	>999	100	.92
Private Psychiatrist	21	1	4	182	100.0	19	0	5	78	94	1.13
Mental Health Centers	21	0	20	260	95.2	19	0	12	78	84	1.35
Family Service Agency	21	0	0	104	23.8	19	0	0	26	31	0.30
Child Guidance Clinic	21	0	1	12	61.9	19	0	1	6	52	0.35
Alcoholics Anonymous	21	0	8	390	76.2	19	0	2	36	51	1.52
Welfare Department	20	0	17.5	390	76.2	19	0	12	200	89	1.22

and the mental health center fourth. Both
groups reported using the Family Service
Agency least often. The reported low
usage of this agency may reflect the absence of such agencies in many of the
counties in which consultation was employed. Chi square statistics were computed in order to determine if reliable
differences in proportions existed between
experimental and control group physicians
who used these various resources. These
results are also presented in Table 11.
No significant differences were observed
between the two groups. We concluded
that the consultation program did not
have a significant effect on physician
use of community resources. As was mentioned in the previous section, physicians
may have relied less on these resources
as they became more confident in treating
patients themselves.

D. *Discussion of Patients' Problems*

It was believed that as experimental
physicians learned about the need for
total patient care and the support that
families and other social systems could
provide the patient, they would report
that they discussed emotional problems of
patients with medical colleagues, local
ministers, patients' family, school personnel, and hospital personnel. Significant differences were obtained between
experimental and control groups only in
the hospital personnel category (x^2=3.65,
df=1, p<.10). Experimental physicians
reported discussing emotional problems

of patients with hospital personnel more
often than any other group. Summarization
of reported usage and significance tests
is given in Table 12.

One can conclude that the consultation program was influential in making
experimental physicians aware of the importance of involving at least one group
in the comprehensive care of the patient.
Experimental physicians may have felt
more comfortable in discussing patient
problems with hospital personnel because
of the trust already acquired in working
with this group over a number of years.
Many experimental physicians had daily
contact with hospital personnel and may
have had more opportunity to discuss emotional problems of patients with them
rather than school personnel, local ministers, patients' family, and medical colleagues.

E. *Time Spent with Patients*

It was believed that experimental
physicians would report spending more time
with psychiatric patients after the physicians began to recognize they could help
alleviate some of the patients' problems
by giving them a little extra attention.
Frequency of change in time spent with
psychiatric patients by experimental and
control groups is reported in Table 13.
Both experimental and control groups reported most often that no change had occurred in the amount of time spent with
psychiatric patients. No significant

Table 12
Discussion of Patients' Problems with Others

	Experimental					Control					
	N	Low	Median	High	Per cent Used	N	Low	Median	High	Per cent Used	x²
Medical Colleagues	21	0	12	>999	76.2	19	0	26	>999	89	1.22
Local Ministers	21	0	6	52	80.9	19	0	2	24	57	2.52
Patients' Family	21	0	100	650	95.2	19	1	52	>999	100	0.93
School Personnel	21	0	2	52	66.7	19	0	2	650	73	0.23
Hospital Personnel	21	0	50	910	80.9	19	0	3	260	52	3.65

Table 13
Time Spent with Psychiatric Patients

	Experimental		Control	
	Frequency	Per cent	Frequency	Per cent
Less Time	4	20	3	16
More Time	5	25	3	16
No Change	11	55	13	68
	20	100	19	100

110

differences were obtained from the chi square analysis ($x^2=.779$, df=2, p>.10).

This finding was not anticipated because Greco (1966), who took a year and one-half from his general practice to attend psychiatric courses, reported that he doubled the amount of time spent with psychiatric patients after returning to his practice. He compensated for the increased amount of time spent discussing emotional problems by varying his fee accordingly, rather than charging a flat fee for an office visit. It is possible that experimental physicians have recognized the need to spend additional time with their emotionally disturbed patients, but have been unable to readjust their office schedules or their fees to allow them more time.

IV.   PROCEDURAL CHECK INFORMATION

The following information was obtained from the interview schedule in order to determine if some of the theoretical assumptions underlying the study were operating to bring about change in physician behavior. The following four reinforcers were identified: communication from a prestigious figure or expert, emotional support from the consultant, escape from an aversive situation of inability to deal with the patient with an emotional problem, and job satisfaction.

A. *Perceived Psychiatric Knowledge of the Consultant*

One of the theoretical assumptions of the study was that experimental physicians would perceive the consultant as prestigious because of his knowledge of mental health concepts. If he were perceived as knowledgeable, it could be assumed from reinforcement theory that experimental physicians would be receptive to a communication from a highly credible communicator and would change their attitudes about patients with emotional problems on the basis of the information delivered by the consultant. Physicians were asked to rank consultants on a scale ranging from very little knowledge to very knowledgeable. Responses for experimental and control groups are presented in Table 14. All 21 of the experimental physicians gave the consultant the highest ranking--very knowledgeable.

This information provides support for the assumption that information delivered by a prestigious figure was a reinforcer operating to bring about behavior change in physicians. Additional support for this assumption was obtained from a ranking of consultant qualities. Experimental physicians were asked to check one or more qualities including academic knowledge, feeling of trust, personality, or relationship as being most important to the consultation experience. Academic knowledge was perceived as most important. Seventeen responses were made in this category. Rankings are presented in Table 15.

Table 14
Perceived Psychiatric Knowledge of the Consultant

	Experimental		Control	
	Frequency	Per cent	Frequency	Per cent
Very Knowledgeable	21	100	17	86.7
Moderately Knowledgeable	0	0	2	13.3
Fairly Knowledgeable	0	0	0	0
Very Little Knowledge	0	0	0	0
	21	100	19	100.0

Table 15
Consultant Qualities

	Experimental Responses
1. Academic Knowledge	17
2. Feeling of Trust in the Consultant	12
3. Personality of the Consultant	11
4. Relationship with the Consultant	11
	51

113

One can conclude from these findings
that the amount of knowledge possessed by
the consultant was an important quality.
Since knowledge is often associated with
being expert or prestigious, it is believed that experimental physicians perceived the consultant as an expert, and
their behavior regarding mental health
practices changed because the information
was delivered by a mental health expert.

B. *Emotional Support from the Consultant*

Another reinforcer operating to
change physician behavior was the emotional support physicians received from
the consultant. It was believed that if
experimental physicians received support
from the consultant, they would feel encouraged to try new or alternate methods
of treating the emotionally disturbed patient. The 21 experimental physicians
were asked to identify what elements from
the consultation process were most helpful
or brought about the most change in the
way they worked with patients. Areas that
physicians named as being most helpful are
ranked in Table 16. Each physician named
one or more areas in which consultation
had been most helpful. Dealing with the
difficult patient was responded to most
frequently, and not enough visits to judge
was named least often. Four of the responses identified emotional support from
the consultant as a helpful aspect of consultation.

Table 16

Significant Material from Consultation

		Experimental Responses
1.	Dealing with difficult patients (psychotic, time-consuming pt., homosexuals, adolescent adj., family problems, marital problems, sexual problems, inadequate personalities, and suicidal patients)	11
2.	Different approach to dealing with mental patients	8
3.	Prescription of drugs for emotional illnesses	6
4.	Dealing with the depressed patient	5
5.	Emotional support from the consultant which led to feelings of increased self-confidence	4
6.	Dealing with the alcoholic	4
7.	Not enough visits to judge	$\frac{2}{41}$

Consultants were also asked what factors of consultation were responsible for bringing about change in physician behavior. The consultants stated their belief that the emotional support they provided physicians in handling some of the current cases, and the encouragement given them to try new or alternate methods of working with the emotionally disturbed patient were helpful.

C.   Escape from an Aversive Situation

Escape from an aversive situation of inability to treat the patient with an emotional problem was another reinforcer operating to change physician behavior. As experimental physicians learned about community resources and specific treatments and skills in working with patients with emotional problems, it was believed they would report feeling more confident than controls. Physicians were asked to check degree of confidence ranging from less confident to definitely more confident. Results of the chi square analysis ($x^2=12.06$, df=2, $p<.01$) provided support that this reinforcer was operating to change behavior. Frequencies of response and percentages for the four categories are reported in Table 17. Experimental physicians checked feeling definitely more confident 33.30 per cent of the time in comparison with no checks in that category from the control group.

One can conclude that increased confidence in working with emotionally dis-

Table 17

Confidence in Working with Psychiatric Patients

	Experimental		Control	
	Frequency	Per cent	Frequency	Per cent
Definitely More Confident	7	33.30	0	0
Somewhat More Confident	11	52.40	19	100
No Different	3	14.30	0	0
Less Confident	0	0.00	0	0
	21	100.00	19	100

117

turbed patients was a reinforcer operating
to change experimental physician behavior.
It is believed that the consultation program provided the experimental physician
with new information and support that en-
abled him to work more effectively with
the emotionally disturbed patient and escape from an aversive one of frustration
and inability to deal with the emotionally
disturbed patient.

D. Job Satisfaction

As experimental physicians acquired
new skills and became more confident in
working with psychiatric patients, it was
believed they would report an increase in
job satisfaction. Results of the chi
square analysis showed the two groups to
be significantly different (x^2=13.05, df=
2, p<.01). Frequencies and percentages
are reported in Table 18. Eighty per cent
of the experimental group, in comparison
to 26 per cent of the control group, reported an increase in job satisfaction.
None of the experimental physicians reported a decrease in job satisfaction,
while 21 per cent of the control group
reported a decrease. The experimental
group reported no change in amount of job
satisfaction 20 per cent of the time,
while the control group reported no change
53 per cent of the time.

These findings lend support to the
belief that job satisfaction was a reinforcer operating to change physician behavior. It is concluded that participation in a consultation program can produce

Table 18

Reported Degree of Job Satisfaction

	Experimental		Control	
	Frequency	Per cent	Frequency	Per cent
Increase	17	80	5	26
Decrease	0	0	4	21
No Change	4	20	10	53
	21	100	19	100

change in experimental physician attitudes about the satisfaction they receive from their jobs.

The present chapter was included for psychiatrists, psychologists, social workers, nurses, and mental health center personnel interested in the computational procedures we used to derive our results. A summary of the results and conclusions from the study are made in the following chapter.

REFERENCES

Brody, M., Golden, M. M. & Lichtman, H. S. Experience with small group seminars for practicing physicians. *American Journal of Psychiatry*, 1965, *122*, 497-500.

Caplan, G. *The theory and practice of mental health consultation*. New York: Basic Books, 1970.

Dorsey, J. R., Matsunaga, G. & Bauman, G. Training public health nurses in mental health. *Archives of General Psychiatry*, 1964, *11*, 214-222.

Enelow, A. J. Can and should we teach psychiatry to practicing nonpsychiatrist physicians? In R. H. Dovenmuehle & J. T. Parmeter (Eds.) *Sixth annual training session for psychiatrist-teachers of practicing physicians, 1965*. Boulder, Colorado; Western Interstate Commission for Higher Education, 1966.

Enelow, A. J. & Adler, L. M. Psychiatric skills and knowledge for the general practitioner. *Journal of the American Medical Association*, 1964, *89*, 91-96.

Forman, L. H., Barnes, R. H., Wilkinson,
      C. B. & McPartland, T. S.   Evaluation
      of teaching efforts with non-
      psychiatric medical practitioners.
      Diseases of the Nervous System, 1964, *25,*
      422-426.
Greco, R. S. & Pittenger, R. A.   *One man's
      practice.*   London: J. P. Lippincott
      Company, 1966.
Norman, E. C. & Forti, T. J.   A study of
      the process and outcome of mental
      health consultation.   *Community Mental
      Health Journal,*   1972, *8* (4),261-270.
Pearson, J. B. & Lee, A.   Questionnaire
      analysis of three seminars, 1967-68.
      In J. B. Pearson (Ed.) *The assessment
      of short-term seminars in psychiatry for
      non-psychiatrist physicians: a progress
      report for the years 1966-68.*   Boulder,
      Colorado: Western Interstate Com-
      mission for Higher Education, 1969.
Pearson, J. B. & Young, T. R.   Question-
      naire analysis of eight seminars
      1963-64.   In J. B. Pearson (Ed.) *The
      analysis of short-term seminars in psychia-
      try for non-psychiatrist physicians: a
      progress report for the years 1963-66.*
      Boulder, Colorado: Western Inter-
      state Commission for Higher Educa-
      tion, 1966.
Pittenger, R. A.   Training physicians in
      the psychologic aspects of medical
      practice.   *Pennsylvania Medical Journal,*
      1962, *65,* 1472-1474.
Schmuck, R. A.   Helping teachers improve
      classroom group processes.   *Journal of
      Applied Behavioral Science,*   1968, *4,* (4),
      401-435.
Stephenson, P. S.   Judging the effective-
      ness of a consultation program to a
      community agency.   *Community Mental
      Health Journal,* 1973, *11,* (3), 253-259.

Zabarenko, L., Pittenger, R. A. & Zaba-
    renko, R. N. *Primary Medical Practice*.
    St. Louis, Missouri: Warren H. Green,
    1968.

5. SUMMARY AND CONCLUSIONS

SUMMARY

Phase One

In retrospect, the first phase (1964-1969) of the program gave us an opportunity to explore a method of delivering information to physicians that we called consultation. It also permitted us to examine the assumption that consultation would be most effective if it were provided on a one-to-one basis in the physician's geographic locale.

During Phase One, we were primarily interested in learning if one physician in each of the western counties of North Carolina could be trained to serve as a mental health resource person to other physicians in his county. Our original goals were modified because many physicians were involved in the planning stages of the program, and asked that the consultant visit

all of them instead of only one physician
in each county. Little attention was
given to goals and evaluation techniques
in the first phase because efforts were
focused on exploring the feasibility of a
new type of educational program to physicians. After four years of experience,
we were able to identify a model of consultation that could be employed by other
consultants. We believed our major ac-
complishment during Phase One was the development of a consultation program in
which physicians demonstrated interest in
learning about mental health concepts.
Although only a postevaluation of the program was conducted, it provided us with
information regarding physicians' perceptions of the consultation program and the
role of the consultant. Physicians also
decreased their referrals for admission
to mental hospitals and changed their drug
prescription patterns after participating
in the program.

Phase Two

The interest of physicians who had
participated in the program, support from
community leaders who had heard of the
program, encouragement from the Department of Mental Health, and available funds
for continuation of the program were factors that influenced us to expand the program, refine our goals, and develop testa-
ble hypotheses during Phase Two. In the
second phase of the program (1970-1973),
we were specifically interested in determining if the mental health consultation
program could produce changes in the

nonpsychiatrist-physician's behavior
toward the emotionally disturbed patient.
Our design for evaluation of the program
included an examination of change in three
areas of physician behavior: knowledge,
attitudes, and skills. Changes in knowledge were assessed by examining scores
on case studies designed to measure psychiatric aspects of illness in the areas
of etiology, clinical impression, diagnostic approach, treatment, and referral
resources. Physician attitudes were assessed by a social distance and social
responsibility scale and responses to the
interview schedule. The social distance
and social responsibility scale was used
to determine if physicians had become more
accepting of the mentally ill person.
Interviews with physicians allowed us to
obtain additional attitudinal measures
regarding physician views of others, perception of the medical certification process, and comfort in working with psychiatric patients. Performance skills of
physicians were determined by examining
referrals to mental hospitals and mental
health centers and responses to the interview questions concerning drug prescription patterns, discussion of patients
with emotional problems, use of community
resources, amount of time spent with psychiatric patients, and types of patients
requiring the most time.

CONCLUSIONS

On the basis of the information we
obtained from the case studies, we concluded that the consultation program did

not produce changes in experimental physicians' knowledge in handling the emotionally ill patient. It is possible that physicians did not receive enough information in the psychiatric aspects of illness regarding etiology, clinical impression, diagnostic approach, treatment approach, and referral resources. Since consultation was not applied consistently because of the many changes in program personnel, this may have been a factor responsible for lack of learning in this area. If consultation was employed two or three times a week for six months or even monthly for two to three years, significant changes might occur in the area of knowledge about mental health approaches in dealing with the emotionally disturbed individual. Zabarenko & Zabarenko (1966) stated that it took two to three years for progress to be seen in physicians who participated in their seminars.

Physician attitude change was observed during the second phase of the program. Experimental physicians reported that they perceived the medical certification process for admitting patients to mental hospitals as less cumbersome after consultation and that they viewed other people with whom they worked differently after consultation. One can conclude that the consultation program was effective in teaching physicians about the procedures for committing patients to the mental hospital and in helping physicians acquire more accepting or tolerant attitudes of nurses, office workers, and other physicians with whom they worked.

No change in attitudes was noted
among physicians in their scores on the
social distance and social responsibility
scale, or in their interview responses in
the area of comfort in working with psychiatric patients. Although one may have
acquired the necessary skills to work with
the emotionally ill and may feel confident
that he can help the emotionally disturbed
individual, there is no guarantee that one
is ever comfortable in the presence of
individuals who are suffering from emotional problems.

During the second phase of the consultation program, changes in performance
skills of physicians were observed in the
areas of drug prescription patterns, referrals to mental hospitals, and discussion
of patients with emotional problems. Unfortunately, no comparisons can be made
regarding drug prescription patterns of
physicians who participated in the consultation program during Phase One and Phase
Two because different questions were asked
during the interviews. We can only assume
from the physicians' verbal reports to the
interviewers that they acquired useful
information regarding medication for the
disturbed patient from the consultants
during both phases of the program.

We believed that consultants during
the 1971-1972 consultation period may have
spent a greater amount of total consultation time discussing the use of appropriate
drugs for the emotionally disturbed patient because physicians reported that
they changed their drug prescription patterns. Changes in physicians' skills were
also noted in the number of referrals to

mental health centers. We believed that
physicians became more confident of their
own skills in handling patients in their
offices and may have referred fewer patients to the mental hospitals. Physicians who participated in the program acquired another skill. They learned about
the importance of involving others in providing total patient care because they
reported they increased their discussion
of patient problems with hospital personnel. Many physicians were in daily contact with hospital personnel and may have
had more opportunity to discuss patients
who had emotional problems with individuals who worked in the hospital.

Reinforcement theory was used to
explain some of the factors responsible
for the learning of mental health concepts. Information was obtained from the
interview schedule which provided support
that four reinforcers were operating to
produce behavior change in physicians.
Consultees reported that they perceived
the consultant as expert, that they received emotional support from the consultant, became more confident in their ability to deal with the mentally ill patient,
and increased in job satisfaction during
consultation.

Since it is generally agreed in our
society that knowledge is associated with
expertness, perception of the consultant
as an expert was an important reinforcer
operating to bring about behavior change
in physicians. It is believed that emotional support from the consultant gave
the physician confidence to handle many
patients who had emotional problems and

try new methods of treating the emotionally disturbed person. As the physician
tried these new behaviors and found them
effective, he began to experience a great
deal of job satisfaction from working with
the individual who had emotional problems.

Although the study was not designed
to measure the verbal behavior of consultants and consultees, it is believed that
verbal reinforcement from the consultant,
when the consultee demonstrated mental
health oriented attitudes and behaviors,
was another factor operating to produce
learning in physicians. The only evidence
that verbal reinforcements were made by
the consultant came from (1) reports by
the consultant that he was supportive to
physicians, (2) statements from the consultees that the support provided by the
consultant gave them confidence to work
with psychiatric patients, and (3) reports
from the consultant that the relationship
with the consultant was one of the most
important parts of the consultation.

Another indication that the second
phase of the program was successful were
the responses to the interview questions
concerning effectiveness, desire to continue consultation or to receive consultation the next year, and recommendation of
the program to other professionals. Nine
of the 21 experimental physicians (42 per
cent) rated the program as excellent and
ten (46 per cent) as good on a four point
scale ranging from poor to excellent.
Two of the physicians said they did not
know how to rate the program. Of the 21
experimental physicians, 95 per cent reported they would like to continue

consultation and 68 per cent of the control physicians indicated they would like to participate in the consultation program the next year. All 21 of the experimental physicians stated they would recommend the program to other professionals.

In summarizing our findings, we examined the reasons why the program may or may not have been successful and made some recommendations that we thought would be useful to psychologists, psychiatrists, social workers, nurses, or other mental health workers who might be interested in pursuing a similar project. These ideas and the activities of the consultants that were pursued after the termination of the evaluation period in 1972 are presented in the next chapter and in Appendix G.

REFERENCES

Zabarenko, L. & Zabarenko, R. N. A suggested method for studying small group seminars in psychiatry. *Journal of Nervous and Mental Diseases,* 1966, *143* (3),239-247.

6. LIMITATIONS, RECOMMENDATIONS, AND INDICATIONS OF SUCCESS

LIMITATIONS AND RECOMMENDATIONS

The major limitations of the consultation program were: (1) lack of well defined goals and the lack of a formal evaluation during Phase One, (2) short period of time evaluation was employed, (3) lack of continuity in the consultation employed in the program, (4) inability of researcher to monitor the content, quality, and amount of consultation, and (5) lack of an accepted theory of consultation in explaining results.

A major limitation of the program from 1964-1969 (Phase One) was the lack of specific goals and methods of achieving them. At the time the program was conceived, the goals were broad and long range. The emphasis was on providing physicians with a type of mental health education program that would interest them in learning about emotional illness and mental health. Little attention was given to the steps

131

necessary to fulfill this goal or to the
formulation of hypotheses that would permit project personnel to evaluate the effectiveness of the program. In 1964, at
the time the project was begun, evaluation
was a term that program administrators
believed in but had little knowledge or
experience in conducting. There were few
studies available to serve as models for
a program evaluation and many program administrators viewed evaluation with ap-
prehension. After four years of experi-
menting with a different type of mental
health education program, the co-directors
of the North Carolina program were interested in learning if their efforts had
been effective. An evaluation of the program was conducted by interviewing physicians who had participated in the program
from 1964 through 1967, although few conclusions regarding effectiveness could be
drawn from only this postevaluation.

During the second phase of the program (1970-1973), goals were identified
but these were general and idealistic.
In planning a future consultation program
it would be helpful if the program director, consultants, and researcher could
agree on a set of short- and long-term
goals prior to initiation of the program.
Ideally, the co-directors, consultants,
and researcher would have a tentative set
of goals which they could modify after
discussing them with the target groups.
Measurement of short- and long-term goals
at six months, one year, and two to five
year intervals could provide feedback to
personnel regarding any changes that would
need to be made in the program.

A second limitation of the second phase of the program (1970-1973) was the short period of time evaluation was conducted. The original evaluation plan was to measure change in physician behavior for a one-year period. Because of the difficulties previously mentioned in maintaining program personnel, consultation occurred for only a ten-month period in six counties and for a five and one-half-month period in one county. Ideally, evaluation would have extended over a two- or three-year period. A nine-month evaluation period may not have been sufficient time to show a great deal of change in physician behavior. Glidewell (1969) states that the most difficult design problem is determining a time interval short enough for program constancy and long enough to demonstrate program effects. It is possible that if consultation had been employed consistently for a year or longer, additional changes in physician behavior would have occurred. Future program directors might wish to compare the effectiveness of weekly consultation for six months with twice-a-month consultation over a one-, two-, or three-year period. Dorsey et al (1964) evaluated a weekly psychiatric consultation program to public health nurses by a psychiatrist, psychiatric social worker, and mental health nurse. At the end of the five-month consultation period, the nurses' understanding of the cases had become more like the consultant; nurses had increased in understanding of individual and family psychodynamics; and a sixty-item rating scale measuring the effects of the conferences showed the greatest effect occurred in nursing knowledge, nursing practices, and attitudes

toward patients. Other studies have not
found such a short training period to be
successful, but perhaps the frequency of
contact rather than length of time the
program was employed was responsible for
its success.

Another limitation was the lack of
continuity of consultation employed because of the resignation of project personnel, the death of one consultant, and
absence of expected state funds for the
expansion of the program to three additional areas of the state. After the
loss of five consultants, the sample size
was reduced and consultation was not employed during the time a new co-director
(psychiatric consultant) was being re-
cruited. The interruption of the consultation program for three months and the
adjustment of physicians to new consultants in two of the areas were important
variables influencing the effectiveness
of the program. One can assume that the
morale of all project staff members was
lowered during these periods of indecision
regarding continuation of the project.
Although all efforts were made to insure
continuity of consultation, it is recommended that in future programs the co-
directors and researcher try to obtain at
least a one year commitment from consultants before employing them. Consultants
in our program had full time jobs at mental health centers, hospitals, or private
practices, and participated in the program only one day a week.

A fourth limitation of the program
was inability of the researcher to monitor the content, quality, and amount of

consultation received by the consultees.
The researcher relied on verbal reports
from the consultants and information
gathered from experimental physicians
during monthly progress meetings regarding the material covered in consultations
and the number of consultation visits.
Since this study was not designed to observe actual consultation between the
consultant and the consultee as in the
Zabarenko and Zabarenko (1966) study,
there were no other means of knowing if
the program goals were being met and if
the consultants were consistent in the
type of information delivered to each
physician. Progress meetings were held
with the consultants regarding content
of the sessions, but the researcher was
not able to control for individual varia-
tions in consultation style. We recommend that prior to the initiation of consultation, consultants provide the researcher and project director with a
detailed description of the type of consultation, content of session, and methods
they intend to use during consultation.
Commitment to the goals of the program
and permission from the consultant and
consultee to observe or record the sessions should be agreed upon prior to the
initiation of the program. Montague &
Taylor (1971) reported on a school consultation program in which consultants
and consultees kept logs of the consultation sessions. This method permitted the
researcher to observe changes in the consultees and in the school children over
a period of time. A similar method could
be used with physicians, nurses, ministers, lawyers, or police groups.

A limitation in the evaluation of
any consultation program is the lack of
an accepted theory of consultation to use
in explaining the results of the program.
This makes generalizing from one program
to the next difficult. Any number of
theories could be used to explain changes
in the consultee group or consultation
process. Mannino & Shore (1971) state
that crisis theory, ecological theory,
and systems theory could supply a useful
orientation to consultation, but currently
none of these has gained acceptance. A
systems approach might be helpful in con-
ceptualizing the consultation process
and enable us to identify some of the
variables that contribute to the effectiveness of the program although mathe-
matical techniques are not available currently to demonstrate cause and effect.
Haylett & Rapoport (1964) state there has
not been time for validation of many of
our working hypotheses either by repeti-
tion or by the experience of other in-
vestigators in a variety of settings.
They believe that until such criteria can
be met there will be no theoretical framework for consultation. In the present
study, reinforcement theory was used to
explain some of the behavior changes in
physicians. The major difficulty with
this theory is identifying which reinforcers are operating to change behavior.
Since many of the studies generated by
this theory have been in the area of verbal reinforcement, it is recommended that
future researchers use tape recordings or
direct observation to determine if verbal
reinforcement that occurs between the
consultant and consultee is effective in
producing behavior change in physicians.

INDICATIONS OF SUCCESS

We have examined limitations of our program and made recommendations to others who may be interested in conducting a similar study. We also believe our program had some strengths because (1) sanction for the program was obtained from institutions and community groups, (2) the target group was involved in the planning of Phase One, (3) consultants had good relationships with their consultees (this fostered learning and permitted the evaluation to be conducted), and (4) consultants were seen as knowledgable, experienced, committed, and having desirable personal characteristics.

Personnel from the Department of Mental Health conceived the idea for the physician consultation program and provided funds for its operation the first year. Because the State Medical Society and local medical societies in the western part of the state were interested in receiving additional mental health resources, they recommended that the program be initiated in the western part of the state. Other institutional sanctions came from the state mental hospital in the western part of the state where the consultant's office was located. During the second phase of the program, two consultants were also employed as directors of the mental health centers in their areas. We believe these ties with state and local institutions contributed to the acceptance and continuation of the program.

Another important factor was the involvement of the consultees in the planning stages of the program during Phase One. We believe these physicians were interested in the program because of their initial support as members of the local medical society and, secondly, their request for the consultants to visit all instead of a few of them.

Consultee evaluations of the consultant during Phase One and Phase Two were positive. Several of the consultees attributed the program's success to the consultants' knowledge of psychiatry, "human" and "down to earth" personalities, and in two instances previous experience as general practitioners.

Perhaps the most important reason the program succeeded was the good relationship that the consultants reported they had with most of their consultees. We believe that an important factor in the physicians' reaction to the program was the cooperation of the physicians during the evaluation of the project. Consultants spent a great deal of time explaining the research part of the program and why the questionnaires and interviews were needed.

SUMMARY

In summary, we believe the type of consultation employed in this study can be an effective method of educating not only physicians, but ministers, lawyers, police, teachers, nurses, and other community groups. We do not see consultation

as replacing lectures, seminars, and work-
shops, but as supplementing a consultation
program. Consultation is costly, but is
seen as a preferred method of education
because it occurs in the consultees' locale and in a one-to-one relationship where
consultees feel free to try new behaviors.
The authors hope that the evaluation of
the physician consultation program conducted in North Carolina will be seen as
only a beginning in evaluation. The limitations and strengths of our program are
recognized, and it is our wish that future
researchers be able to benefit from our
experiences over the past ten years and
the recommendations that have grown out of
them. We hope that researchers will de-
vote more attention to the identification
and measurement of program goals, attempt
to develop and refine current instruments
used to assess program effectiveness, and
continue to test hypotheses which may be
used for building a theory of consultation.

REFERENCES

Dorsey, J. R., Matsunaga, G. & Bauman, G.
    Training public health nurses in men-
    tal health. *Archives of General Psychia-
    try*, 1964, *11*,214-222.
Glidewell, J. C. Research problems in
    community psychology. In A. J. Bind-
    man & A. D. Spiegel (Eds.) *Perspec-
    tives in community mental health*. Chicago:
    Aldine, 1969.
Haylett, C. H. & Rapoport, L. Mental
    health consultation. In L. Bellak
    (Ed.) *Handbook of community psychiatry*.
    New York: Grune and Stratton, 1964.

Mannino, F. V. & Shore, M. F.   Consulta-
    tion research in mental health and
    related fields.   Public Health Mono-
    graph No. 79, Public Health Service
    Publication No. 2122, U. S. Depart-
    ment of Health, Education, and Wel-
    fare, U. S. Government Printing Of-
    fice, Washington, D. C., 1971.
Montague, Ernest K. & Taylor, Elaine N.
    *Preliminary handbook on procedures for eval-
    uating mental health.*   Indirect Service
    Programs in Schools (Prepared for
    NIMH Health Services and Mental Health
    Administration, Department of Health,
    Education, and Welfare) by Human Re-
    sources Research Organization, Alexan-
    dria, Virginia, 1971.
Zabarenko, L. & Zabarenko, R. N.   A sug-
    gested method for studying small
    group seminars in psychiatry.   *Journal
    of Nervous and Mental Diseases,* 1966, *143*
    (3),239-247.

APPENDICES

APPENDIX A

MAP OF COUNTIES THAT PARTICIPATED IN THE CONSULTATION PROGRAM
Phase I 1964-1969   Phase II 1970-1973

Broughton Hospital

Region I (Western)

NORTH CAROLINA

Region II (North Central) John Umstead Hospital

Region III (South Central) Dorothea Dix Hospital

Region IV (Eastern) Cherry Hospital

+ = Consultation employed in the 5 western counties, 1964-1967
■ = Consultation employed in the 3 eastern counties, 1968-1969
△ = Consultation and evaluation in 6 counties for 10 months--6/71-6/72
● = Consultation and evaluation in 10 counties for 3 months--6/71-8/71
⧉ = Consultation and evaluation employed for 5½ months from 6/71-8/71, and from 12/71-2/72

143

APPENDIX B
DRUG QUESTIONNAIRE

	Average Dose	Dose Range	For which Symptoms, Disorders
Librium	___	___	___
Valium	___	___	___
Serax	___	___	___
Meprobamate (Equanil, Miltown)	___	___	___
Tybamate (Tybatran, Solacen)	___	___	___
Vistaril, Atarax	___	___	___
Deprol	___	___	___
Thorazine	___	___	___
Vesprin	___	___	___
Sparine	___	___	___
Mellaril	___	___	___
Prolixin, Permitil	___	___	___
Trilafon	___	___	___
Compazine (other than for nausea)	___	___	___

DRUG QUESTIONNAIRE CONTINUED

	Average Dose	Dose Range	For which Symptoms, Disorders
Stelazine	___	___	___
Taractan	___	___	___
Navane	___	___	___
Haldol	___	___	___
Tofranil	___	___	___
Elavil	___	___	___
Norpramin, Pertofrane	___	___	___
Aventyl	___	___	___
Vivactil	___	___	___
Etrafon, Triavil	___	___	___
Ritalin	___	___	___
Barbiturates and other hypnotics for daytime sedation (specify which, when, dosage)	___	___	___
Amphetamines (specify which, when, dosage)	___	___	___

What medications do you use I.M. and I.V. in the emergency room to control agitation (dosage and route)?

_____

Are there any combinations of the above drugs which you use frequently?

_____
_____

_____
What percentage of your patients at one
time or another have received any of the
above mentioned drugs? _____
What drugs do you use in treating alcoholism?

_____
What drugs do you use in treating child-
hood behavior disorders?

_____
_____

APPENDIX C
QUESTIONNAIRE

INSTRUCTIONS

Name: _____
Length of time in practice: _____
Type of professional training: _____
_____
Number of years of professional training:
_____
Previous training or experience in Mental
Health: _____
_____

Instructions

The following brief histories are given in
order for you to respond to your clinical
impression, diagnostic approach, suspected
etiology, treatment approach, and community resource assistance. In each case,
we would like you to consider being con-
fronted with the problem in the context of
your usual and routine working day. We

would expect different specialists (for example, surgeons and psychiatrists) to respond differently. In this way, there are no right or wrong answers. We are interested in how you perceive the situation from the brief information given you. Although the questions are couched in terms of organic illness or emotional illness, you would not be expected in your own practice to assume a psychiatric bias toward the problem unless, possibly, you were a psychiatrist. In essence, we would like you to assume your own individual orientation toward the problem. With that in mind, please rank in order of your own preference, No.1 for your first choice, No.2 for second choice, No.3 for third choice, and No.4 for your least preferable choice.

> Example: Carrots as your
>   favorite vegetable

> No.4 - least preferred
> No.2 - second best
> No.1 - most preferred
> No.3 - third best

A.   CASE STUDIES

Vignette No.1

A 45-year old white male engineer suffered coronary thrombosis one year ago. Previously he was physically active, busy, and assertive. He now complains of recurrent chest pain brought on by either physical or emotional stress. He appears depressed and states that curtailment of his activities and work makes his life dull and meaningless.

A. Immediate Clinical Impression: (most likely problem)
    _____Depressive reaction
    _____Coronary insufficiency producing angina
    _____Depressive reaction secondarily producing coronary insufficiency
    _____Coronary insufficiency with secondary depressive reaction

B. Immediate Assessment: (initial diagnostic approach)
    _____Complete cardiac workup--physical examination, ECG, catheterization, etc.
    _____Determine cardiac status and reassure patient that he can be rehabilitated
    _____Interviews with patients to determine conflicts responsible for his emotional reactions
    _____Interview with patient to help him understand the disability so he may react more appropriately to his condition

C. Immediate Impression of Etiology or Understanding of the Problem:
    _____Physical symptoms impairing patient's life style which in turn leads to his depression
    _____Loss of interest, self-esteem, and fear of death
    _____Depression producing stress which in turn causes angina
    _____Circulatory impairment producing symptoms

D. Treatment and Disposition: (most
    likely treatment approach)
    _____Frequent interviews with patient
           to help him better cope and adapt
           to his decreased physical func-
           tioning
    _____Prescribing appropriate physical
           exercises and medications to in-
           crease cardiac function and med-
           cations to ameliorate depression
    _____Reassurance, medications for pain
           relief and depression
    _____Coronary vasodilating drugs and
           possible arterial graft

E. Other Community Resources for As-
    sistance:
    _____Refer to specialized medical cen-
           ter for cardiac surgery
    _____Local mental health professionals
    _____One of your colleagues very adept
           in treating this particular ill-
           ness
    _____Minister-counselor

Vignette No.2

A 35-year old Negro laborer is seen in
your office complaining of low-back pain
sustained from a job injury. In response
to your questions concerning his symptoms,
he is somewhat belligerent and refuses to
actively cooperate in your examination.
He was insistent that you justify his absence from work to his employer.

A. Immediate Clinical Impression: (most
    likely problem)
    _____Malingering

_____Expected physical illness because
       of this man's occupation and
       physical stature
_____Emotional reaction of a man to
       his demeaning job and second
       class status producing physical
       symptoms
_____Physical illness with concomitant
       emotional reaction to pain and
       discomfort

B. Immediate Assessment: (initial diag-
    nostic approach)
    _____Minimal diagnostic procedures so
           patient's manipulation will not
           be reinforced
    _____Physical examination and explore
           with him his concern about his
           condition
    _____Appropriate physical examination
           to determine specific disease
           entity
    _____Explore with him his feelings
           about his job, life status and
           his superiors

C. Your Understanding of the Physical and
    Emotional Causes of the Problem:
    _____Due to his physical condition and
           suffering, he is worried about
           his health, loss of job and in-
           come, family status, etc.
    _____Incapacitating physical condition
    _____Conversion of emotional conflicts
           into physical symptoms
    _____Hostile attitude because he is
           fearful the doctor will expose
           his malingering

D. Treatment and Disposition: (most like-
    ly treatment approach)

_____Symptomatic relief and reas-
surance that he will recover

_____Emotional support and counseling;
encourage patient to continue
work

_____Refuse treatment of physical
symptoms; firmly direct patient
to return to work

_____Bed rest, analgesics, and seda-
tives for amelioration of symptoms

E. Community Resources for Assistance:
(persons or agencies other than yourself who could be of help with the
problem)

_____Patient's employer--personnel
director, foreman, etc.

_____Local mental health center

_____Vocational rehabilitation for
job retraining

_____None - Interference from other
agencies will only serve to
further his incapacitation

Vignette No.3

A 16-year old girl is brought to your office by her parents with the following
symptoms: headache, loss of appetite,
vague abdominal pain, and sleeplessness.
They state that she is rebellious, she has
lost interest in school, and does not get
along with her family. They are angry
with her and are seeking help for the physical symptoms.

A. Immediate Clinical Impression: (most
likely problem)

_____Primarily emotional and secondary
physical symptoms
_____Organic illness: i.e., infec-
tious, metabolic, hormonal, etc.
_____Family conflicts are causing the
symptoms
_____She is in trouble: i.e., drugs,
pregnancy, bad grades, etc.

B.   Initial Assessment: (diagnostic approach)
_____Interview of patient alone
_____Complete physical examination
and laboratory evaluation
_____ Interview with parents and patient together
_____ Obtain history from parents and
girl and do physical examination
to reassure family

C.   Immediate Impression of Etiology or
Understanding of the Problem:
_____Reaction to parents' pressure to
perform according to their expectations
_____ Physical illness causing emotional
symptoms
_____ Adolescent adjustment reaction
_____ She is being influenced by other
rebellious teenagers and got
into trouble

D.   Treatment and Disposition: (most likely treatment approach)
_____Hospitalization and consultation
with surgeon
_____Frequent interviews with girl
alone and prescription for mild
tranquilizers
_____Frequent interviews with patient
and parents together

_____Appropriate treatment of physical illness

E. Other Community Resources for Assistance: (persons or agencies other than yourself who could be of help with the problem)
_____School counselor
_____Minister trained in counseling
_____Welfare Department caseworker
_____Local mental health professionals

Vignette No.4

A 28-year old white female is seen in the Emergency Room with symptoms of mental confusion, loss of memory, disorientation for place and time, and fearfulness. Her agitation is so great that she requires restraining. The symptoms began two days ago and progressively worsened. Her physical examination was normal other than markedly dilated pupils, tachycardia, and mild elevation of systolic blood pressure.

A. Immediate Clinical Impression: (most likely problem)
_____Acute psychotic reaction, probably schizophrenia
_____Acute brain injury due to cerebral vascular accident
_____Acute toxic organic brain syndrome with delirium
_____Hysterical reaction with conversion symptoms

B. Initial Assessment: (diagnostic approach)
_____Complete history from family

regarding exposure to toxins, drugs, alcohol, family history, etc.

_____Benign neglect to avoid being manipulated by the patient

_____Complete neurological examination

_____Tranquilization of patient, and determine from family as well as patient precipitating circumstances leading to psychotic reaction

C. Immediate Impression of Etiology or Understanding of the Problem:

_____Mental state acutely impaired by psychotic process

_____Mental state acutely impaired by toxic disease process

_____Mental state is functional and the process is emotionally induced

_____Mental state acutely impaired by change in gross organic structure of the brain

D. Treatment and Disposition: (most likely treatment approach)

_____Minor tranquilizers and hospitalize in quiet room

_____Major tranquilization: i.e., phenothiazines, and consider immediate hospitalization in psychiatric hospital

_____Treatment of the toxic condition once the specific toxin is determined

_____Neurological or neurosurgical consultation

E. Other Community Resources for Assistance: (persons or agencies other

158   CONSULTATION-EDUCATION

than yourself who could be of help
with the problem)
_____ Local mental health center
_____ Refer to medical center
_____ Minister trained in counseling
_____ One of your colleagues adept in
        treating neurological conditions

Vignette No.5

A 42-year old white woman, mother of two
grown children and wife of a salesman,
is seen in your office complaining of severe headaches. The headaches are described as severe, bilateral, pounding in
character, producing nausea and sleeplessness. She has been to other doctors who
have tried many different medications which
were of little or no help.

A. Immediate Clinical Impression: (most
    likely problem)
    _____ Family conflicts are causing the
          symptoms
    _____ Depressed middle-aged woman
    _____ Organic disease - infectious,
          metabolic, neoplastic, vascular,
          etc.
    _____ Hysterical middle-aged woman

B. Initial Assessment: (diagnostic ap-
    proach)
    _____ Combined interview with husband
          and wife
    _____ Complete physical evaluation in-
          cluding skull x-rays and EEG
    _____ Physical examination and trial
          of tranquilizers
    _____ Exploration of precipitating

events and conflicts producing
symptoms

C. Immediate Impression of Etiology or
Understanding of the Problem:
_____Inadequate personality
_____Patient is victim of organic
          disease
_____Depressive reaction mixed with
          tension and anxiety
_____Anxiety resulting from her loss
          of status in the family

D. Treatment and Disposition: (most
likely treatment approach)
_____Encourage patient to discuss
          events leading to symptom devel-
          opment and prescribe tranquil-
          izers
_____Appropriate treatment of the or-
          ganic disease
_____Confronting the patient with the
          fact that she is responsible for
          her own symptoms and give firm
          directions
_____Marital counseling with husband
          and wife together

E. Other Community Resources for As-
sistance: (persons or agencies other
than yourself who could be of help with
the problem
_____Local hospital for neurologic
          evaluation
_____Minister trained in marriage
          counseling
_____Fellow professional colleague who
          has the knack for dealing with
          this type of patient
_____Local mental health professionals

B. SOCIAL DISTANCE AND SOCIAL RESPONSIBILITY ATTITUDE SCALE

The following statements express how some people feel about life in general and about mental illness. Please indicate whether you agree or disagree with each of these sayings by placing a (1) if you strongly agree, (2) if you agree, (3) if you are neutral, (4) if you disagree, and (5) if you strongly disagree, in the space provided to the left of each statement.

Response Categories: 1. Strongly Agree
                         2. Agree
                         3. Neutral
                         4. Disagree
                         5. Strongly Disagree

_____The family and friends of a mentally ill person need mental health education.

_____I would feel partially responsible if a member of my favorite club became mentally ill.

_____In spite of our best efforts, there is very little which we can do to prevent mental illness.

_____Those who live in communities from which the mentally ill come need to be educated about mental illness.

_____People living in communities from which mentally sick people come are partially responsible for their breakdown.

_____I would feel partially responsible if a member of my family had a serious mental breakdown.

_____I would be willing to sponsor a person who had been mentally ill for

membership in my favorite club or
society.

_____If I owned an empty lot beside my
house, I would be willing to sell
it to a former mental hospital patient.

_____I would be willing to room with some-
one who had been a patient in a mental hospital.

_____I can imagine myself falling in love
with a person who had been mentally
ill.

_____We should strongly discourage our
children from marrying anyone who
has been mentally ill.

_____I wouldn't hesitate to work with some-
one who had been mentally ill.

_____I would be opposed to having a person
who had been in a mental hospital
teach my children.

_____If I owned an apartment house and
lived there, I would not hesitate
to rent an apartment to a person
discharged from a mental hospital.

_____If I could do the job and the pay were
right, I wouldn't mind working in
a mental hospital.

APPENDIX D
INTERVIEW SCHEDULE

EXPERIMENTAL

Name: Date:

Introduction: I'm Carole Vacher, a researcher with the Physician Consultation
Project. I'm here today to ask your opinion about the consultation program. Has
it been of use to you? Has it influenced
your practice? What kind of program do
you think it was? How would you change
it?

All responses are confidential and no
names will be used in the study.

1. Do you have any of the following resources in your community?

Resource	Have you used?	No. of times since consultation
Public Health Clinic	_____	_____
Private Psy- chiatrists	_____	_____
Mental Health Clinic	_____	_____
Family Service Agency	_____	_____
Child Guidance Clinic	_____	_____
Alcoholics Anonymous	_____	_____
Welfare Depart- ment	_____	_____

Are you more or less inclined to use these resources as a result of consultation? Yes___ No___

Are you satisfied with the mental health resources in your community? Yes___No___

2. As a result of the consultation do you find that you discuss problems with any of the following?

	Yes	No	No. of times since consultation
Medical Col- leagues	___	___	_____
Local Ministers	___	___	_____
Members of the Pa- tient's Family	___	___	_____
School Personnel	___	___	_____
Hospital Personnel	___	___	_____

3. Have you noticed any difference in the psychotropic medicines you are prescribing now as compared to before consultation? Yes___No___. Can you give me some quantifiable answer that would reflect that change?_____

_____

_____

Have you noticed any change in the type of drugs you prescribe to the severely disturbed patient? Yes___No___Type_____
Dosage_____

Have you noticed any change in the type of drugs you prescribe to the mildly disturbed psychiatric patient? Yes___No___Type_____
Dosage_____

Have you noticed any change in the type of drug or drugs you prescribe to the nonpsychiatric patient who complains of nervousness? Yes___No___Type_____Dosage_____

How about barbiturates?_____
How about major tranquilizers?_____
How about the minor tranquilizers?_____

If you have noticed a change in the way you are prescribing drugs, what do you think is responsible for the change?

                          Approximately what
                          per cent of these
                          have influenced
                             the change?

Journals_____   _____
Pharmaceutical
   Representatives_____   _____
Consultants_____   _____
Other Physicians_____   _____

4. Have you noticed any changes in the kinds of patients you like to work with as a result of consultation?

What types?_____
          _____
          _____
          _____

Are there certain patients you prefer not to work with as a result of consultation?
_____

Are there certain patients you feel more comfortable with since consultation?_____
_____
_____

5. How do you feel about working with psychiatric patients now as compared to before consultation?

Definitely more confident_____
Somewhat more relaxed _____
No difference_____
Less competent_____

6. Have you noticed any changes in the amount of time you spend with certain patients now as compared to before consultation?

(a) Do you see more or fewer patients?
     More___Fewer___What per cent?_____

(b) Which patients do you see for longer periods of time?_____
_____

If (b) answered incompletely, ask (c) What types of problems take more of your time?
_____

If answer still incomplete, suggest the following:

	Do you see?	How many?
Dying Patient	_____	_____
Alcoholic Patient	_____	_____
Aged	_____	_____
Pregnant Teenager	_____	_____
Menopausal Women	_____	_____
Children	_____	_____
Suicidal Patients	_____	_____

7. What per cent of the people you formerly referred to the mental health center, psychiatrists, mental hospital, or other community resource can you now serve at your office?

	Per cent
Mental Health Center	_____
Psychiatrists	_____
Mental Hospital	_____
Others	_____

8. Do you find the medical certification process for admitting patients to the mental hospital too cumbersome? Yes___ No___ Do you feel consultation has made it easier to refer patients to the mental health center or mental hospital? Yes___ No___ If yes, how was consultation helpful?

_____

_____

9. Have you noticed any increase_____ or decrease_____in job satisfaction as a

result of consultation?_____
_____
_____

10. Have you noticed any change in the
way you view other people since consultation? Yes___No____

                                    In what
                                     way?___

Examples: Other Phy-
              sicians   _____   _____
           Patients   _____   _____
           Nurses   _____   _____
           Office Staff_____   _____
           Family of
              Patients   _____   _____

11. How many times did the consultant
visit with you? 5___10___15___20___More___

12. Can you recall any especially significant material from consultation that has
helped in your day-to-day practice?_____
_____
_____

13. How much did you feel you needed consultation? Considerable___ Fair amount____
Occasionally___Very little____

14. How do you perceive the consultant as
to the amount of psychiatric knowledge possessed?

Very knowledgeable about psychiatric problems _____
Moderately knowledgeable about psychiatric
   problems_____

Fairly knowledgeable about psychiatric
   problems_____
Very little knowledge about psychiatric
   problems_____

15. If you feel the consultation relationship has been helpful, can you identify what it was that was most helpful or
brought about the most change in you or
the way you work with patients?_____
_____
_____
_____

(Suggestions if he cannot identify factors
that may have been responsible)

Consultant's personality   _____
Relationship with consultant   _____
Feeling of trust in consultant_____
Academic knowledge possessed   _____
   by the consultant
Others   _____

Would you like to continue consultation?
Yes___No___

16. Would you recommend consultation to
others? Yes___No___
Would you recommend for general practi-
tioners_____, physician specialists_____,
nurses_____, others_____?

17. How would you rate the consultation
program? Excellent_____Good_____Fair_____
Poor_____. If you could change the consultation program, what would you do differently?_____
_____

18. How would you rate the research component of the consultation program?
Excellent_____Good_____Fair_____Poor_____

If you could change it, what would you do differently?_____

_____

_____

Interviewer's comments: Was the doctor?
            Very cooperative   _____
            Fairly cooperative   _____
            Neutral   _____
            Somewhat hostile   _____
            Very hostile   _____

INTERVIEW SCHEDULE (Continued)
CONTROL

Name: Date:

Introduction: I'm Carole Vacher, a researcher with the Physician Consultation
Project. I'm interested in knowing if you
have noticed any changes in your practice
within the past six months? For instance,
this July compared with last December?

1. Do you have any of the following resources in your community?

Resource	Have you used?	No. of times during past six months?
Public Health Clinic	_____	_____
Private Psy- chiatrists	_____	_____
Mental Health Clinic	_____	_____
Family Service Agency	_____	_____
Child Guidance Clinic	_____	_____
Alcoholics Anonymous	_____	_____
Welfare Department	_____	_____

Have you noticed any increase in the frequency with which you have used these resources during the past six months?
Yes____No____

Are you satisfied with the mental health
resources in your community? Yes____No____

2. Do you discuss patients you suspect as having emotional problems or just problems in general with any of the following?

	Yes	No	No. of times within past six months?
Medical Colleagues	___	___	_____
Local Ministers	___	___	_____
Members of Patient's Family	___	___	_____
School Personnel	___	___	_____
Hospital Personnel	___	___	_____

3. Have you noticed any differences in the psychotropic medicines you are prescribing now as compared to six months ago? Can you give me some quantifiable answer that would reflect that change?

_____

_____

Have you noticed any change in the type of drugs you prescribe to the severely disturbed psychiatric patient? Yes___ No___Type_____Dosage_____

Have you noticed any change in the type of drugs you prescribe to the mildly disturbed psychiatric patient? Yes___No___ Type_____Dosage_____

Have you noticed any change in the type of drug or drugs you prescribe to the non-psychiatric patient who complains of nervousness? Yes___No___Type_____Dosage_____

How about barbiturates?_____
How about major tranquilizers?_____
How about the minor tranquilizers?_____

If you have noticed a change in the way
you are prescribing drugs, what do you
think is responsible for the change?

Approximately what per cent of these have
influenced the change?

Journals   _____
Pharmaceutical Representatives_____
Consultants   _____
Other Physicians   _____

4. Have you noticed any change in the
kinds of patients you like to work with
over the past six months? What types?

_____

_____

Are there certain patients you prefer not
to work with now as compared to six months
ago?_____

_____

_____

Are there certain patients you feel more
comfortable with now as compared to six
months ago?_____

_____

_____

5. How do you feel about working with
psychiatric patients now as compared to
six months ago?

Definitely more confident_____
Somewhat more confident _____
No difference_____
Less competent_____

6. Have you noticed any changes in the
amount of time you spend with certain patients now in comparison with six months
ago?

(a) Do you see more or fewer patients?
More_____Fewer_____What per cent_____

(b) Which patients do you see for longer
periods of time?_____

If (b) answered incompletely, ask (c).
What types of problems take more of your
time?_____

If answer still incomplete, suggest the
following:

	Do you see?	How many?
Dying Patient	_____	_____
Alcoholic Patient	_____	_____
Aged	_____	_____
Pregnant Teenager	_____	_____
Menopausal Women	_____	_____
Children	_____	_____
Suicidal Patients	_____	_____

7. Do you find the medical certification
process for admitting patients to the mental hospital too cumbersome? Yes___No___

Do you feel referring patients to the mental health center or mental hospital has
been any easier within the past six months?
Yes___No___. If yes, what factors do you
see as responsible?_____
_____

8. Have you noticed any increase or decrease in job satisfaction within the past
six months? Increase_____Decrease_____

If an increase, what factors have contributed to the change?_____
_____

9. Have you noticed any change in the way you view other people within the past six months? Yes___No___

In what
way?

Examples: Other
           Physicians _____   _____
           Patients   _____   _____
           Nurses   _____   _____
           Office Staff _____   _____
           Family of
           Patients   _____   _____

10. Would you like to receive consultation this year? Yes___No___

11. How much do you feel you need consultation? Considerable_____Fair amount_____ Occasionally_____Very little_____

12. How do you perceive the consultant in your region as to amount of psychiatric knowledge possessed?

Very knowledgeable about psychiatric problems_____
Moderately knowledgeable about psychiatric problems_____
Fairly knowledgeable about psychiatric problems_____
Very little knowledge about psychiatric problems_____

13. How would you rate the research component of the consultation program?

Excellent_____ Good_____Fair_____Poor_____
If you could change it, what would you do
differently?_____

_____

Interviewer's Comments: Was the doctor:
            Very cooperative _____
            Fairly cooperative_____
            Neutral _____
            Somewhat hostile_____
            Very hostile_____

I Phase

1963
Planning for a mental health education-consultation program by N. C. Dept. of Mental Health.

1964
Implementation of program in counties in western N. C.

1965-1966-1967
Operation of program in western N. C.

1968-1969
Expansion of program to eastern N. C. Evaluation of program in western N. C.

II Phase

1970
Expansion of program to three additional areas of the state. Recruitment of new personnel.

1971-Spring
Implementation of consultation program in five areas of N. C.

1. Design for program evaluation
   a. Selection of experimental and control groups
   b. Validation of instruments
   c. Administration of questionnaires to experimental and control physicians

1971-Summer
Resignation of project personnel.

1971-Fall
Program limited to three areas of state.

1971-Winter
Validation of instruments.

1972-Summer
Data Collection
1. Interviews
2. Administration of post-evaluation questionnaire. End of evaluation of Phase II.

1972-Fall - December 1973
Expansion or continuation of consultation program. No evaluation.

APPENDIX F
PROCEDURES USED TO ESTABLISH RELIABILITY
OF CASE STUDIES AND SOCIAL DISTANCE
AND SOCIAL RESPONSIBILITY SCALE

*Procedures Used to Establish Reliability of Case
Studies*

An iterative process with two steps
was followed in the evaluation of appro-
priateness of case study items for the
present study. First, the coefficient of
concordance was used to determine agreement among judges' rankings of the ap-
propriateness of alternatives. Coefficients of concordance were obtained separately for the pre- and post-tests. In
order to be included in the scale, an
average coefficient of concordance of .60
over pre- and postadministrations was assumed to represent substantial agreement
between judges. The rationale for this
step was that if expert judges could agree
among themselves as to the rank order of
desirability of the four alternatives presented with each case study item on two
separate occasions, then the item measured
aspects of the process followed in handling individuals with mental illness which

would be accepted by experts in the field of mental health. This would also provide a ranking of the desirability of each of the four alternatives to the five content areas of etiology, clinical impression, diagnostic impression, treatment, and referral resource.

The second stage was concerned with providing evidence that the judges were internally consistent from one ranking session to another. Rank order correlations were obtained for each judge on his pre- and postrankings of alternatives for each item. An average pre-post rank order correlation of .50 was selected as the criterion level for retaining judges in the analysis.

This evaluation procedure resulted in two of the judges being dropped because of inconsistent pre-post rankings. The evaluation process was carried out separately for each of the 25 items in the instrument. The final iteration of the item selection procedure left 14 items and seven judges which met the joint criteria of consistency between judges on the two administrations and consistency within judges.

An item by judge two-way analysis of variance was conducted to determine if homogeneity of rankings could be established across judges and across items. Analyses were conducted on the Spearman rank order correlation coefficients and transformed into Fisher Z's. Nonsignificant F's for both support the contention that the 14 items represented a homogeneous and reliable scale. Based upon these results, it was concluded that this set of judges was consistent over time and consistent in responses to items.

Procedures Used to Establish the Reliability of the Social Distance and Social Responsibility Scale

In determining the internal consistency of the social responsibility and social distance scale, Winer's* (1962, p. 128) analysis of variance approach for estimated reliability of measurements was applied to the judges' individual question responses. The judges were highly consistent in their responses at pretest (r= .944) and post-test (r=.889). Further, a Pearson Product Moment Correlation of the judges' prescale scores obtained in February 1971, and the judges' postscale scores obtained in May 1972, showed a strong relationship (r=.774), thus indicating a high degree of stability among the items in the social distance and social responsibility scale. However, an inspection of the mean total scale scores for the validating group of judges revealed a shift of approximately six points in a negative direction from the first to second administrations (26.33 to 32.22). This finding was difficult to reconcile with the observed high reliability within the pre- and postadministrations and between the administrations. A discussion

*Winer, B. J.   *Statistical principles in experimental design.*   New York: McGraw-Hill Book Company, 1962.

with the validating judges in the Department of Mental Health revealed that the post-test administration coincided with a particularly hectic and stressful period for most of the judges which may have resulted in the less favorable attitude being elicited. It is also possible that psychiatrists may have resented taking the questionnaire the second time. During the first administration judges may have tended to give the expected or "most desirable" answer. It was decided that the high consistency of judges did suggest that the pretest administration would be more representative of the type of attitudes held by experts in mental health toward the emotionally disturbed.

APPENDIX G
PROGRAM ACTIVITIES FOLLOWING
THE 1971-1972 EVALUATION PERIOD

After the grant period ended, consultation continued in three areas of the state. The consultant in the western part of the state involved other mental health professionals in a consultation program to physicians on emergency room duty at local hospitals in his area. Physicians in two counties who had previously received individual consultation began contacting social workers, nurses, or psychologists from the mental health center who were on call to help them plan for individuals who came to the emergency room during a crisis period. Mental health center personnel often received calls from physicians regarding alcoholics, attempted suicides, and individuals reacting to an emotional situation with a physical complaint. In some instances mental health center personnel would provide physicians with further diagnostic services if the patient were admitted to the general hospital or help them admit a patient to the state mental hospital or refer them for out-patient treatment at the local mental

health center. In the two counties which
did not have psychiatric resources, physicians regularly contacted mental health
center personnel approximately six times
per week regarding patients with mental
health problems. In one of the counties
a psychiatrist was employed by the mental
health clinic to provide case consultation
to physicians. In addition to the emergency room consultation in two of the
counties and consultation by the psychiatrist in another county, the area was
awarded a five-year Appalachian Regional
Development Grant for continuation of consultation in all the counties who had
originally received consultation services.

The consultant in the central area
of the state extended his program to group
consultation in addition to the client and
consultee centered consultation employed
during the 1971-1972 evaluation period.
The mental health center in his area provided funds for continuation of the program and helped him organize weekly lun-
cheon meetings with physicians. During
these luncheons physicians discussed mental health problems that they had identified as difficult or viewed mental health
films dealing with specific mental health
problems.

In the eastern part of the state consultation continued to be employed with
physicians on an individual basis, and
some control physicians who participated
in the evaluation period also began receiving consultation. During December
1973, the consultant contacted the local
mental health center regarding continuation of the consultation program, but

funds were not available to support the
program in the eastern area.

The consultation program that began
with only one psychiatric consultant in
1964 was expanded to five areas of the
state in 1971 and has continued in three
areas of the state. Social workers, psychologists, and nurses at the mental
health centers in two of the areas are
regularly contacted by some physicians
regarding mental health problems.

In retrospect, we believe that the
program continued to expand in two areas
of the state because the consultant was
affiliated with the local mental health
center. Personnel in both mental health
centers became involved in the project
and continued their activities. The mental health center had funds to support
personnel to provide consultation and was
seen by the consultees and other community
groups as a resource they could utilize
when future consultation was needed. In
the eastern area the consultant did not
base his operations from the mental health
center, and he had neither funds nor personnel from the mental health center to
continue the consultation activities he
began.

INDEX

188   INDEX